Collins

How I Feel

40 wellbeing activities for kids

Becky Goddard-Hill
Assia Ieradi

This book is dedicated to my precious Pocket People who always take such beautiful care of my feelings.

And with my heartfelt thanks to Michelle, Gillian, James and Assia for helping create this gorgeous book.

Published by Collins
An imprint of HarperCollins*Publishers*
Westerhill Road
Bishopbriggs
Glasgow
G64 2QT

HarperCollins*Publishers*
Macken House, 39/40 Mayor Street Upper,
Dublin 1, D01 C9W8, Ireland

collins.co.uk

First published 2023

Illustrations by Assia Ieradi

Publisher: Michelle I'Anson
Project manager: Gillian Bowman
Design: James Hunter and Kevin Robbins
Cover: Assia Ieradi and James Hunter
Production: Ilaria Rovera

A catalogue record for this book is available from the British Library.

ISBN: 9780008649975

Printed in Great Britain by Bell and Bain Ltd, Glasgow.

10 9 8 7 6 5 4 3 2

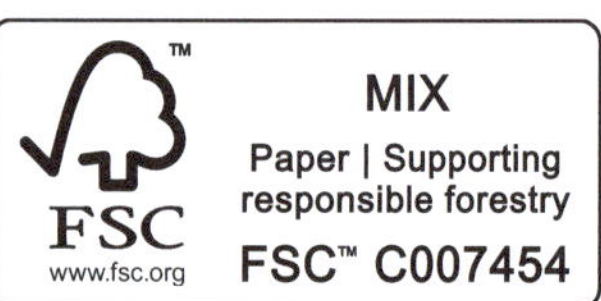

This book contains FSC™ certified paper and other controlled sources to ensure responsible forest management.

For more information visit: www.harpercollins.co.uk/green

Introduction

Some feelings are brilliant.

If you feel excited, it might be because it's your birthday or because Gran is coming to stay.

Some feelings are difficult.

If you feel sad, it might be because your pet is poorly, or you didn't get asked to play.

It is useful to think about your feelings. They give you lots of important information and can help you decide what to do.

It also helps to let your feelings out. If they get stuck inside, they can make you feel worse.

This book will show you how to talk about your feelings more easily and ways to feel happier, kinder, calmer and braver.

For grown-ups

It is hugely beneficial for children to learn to talk about their feelings and find positive ways to manage and express them. Sometimes though, it can make them feel emotional and they may need your support, so just let them know you are there if they need you and that it's always okay for them to talk to you about how they feel.

Meet the characters

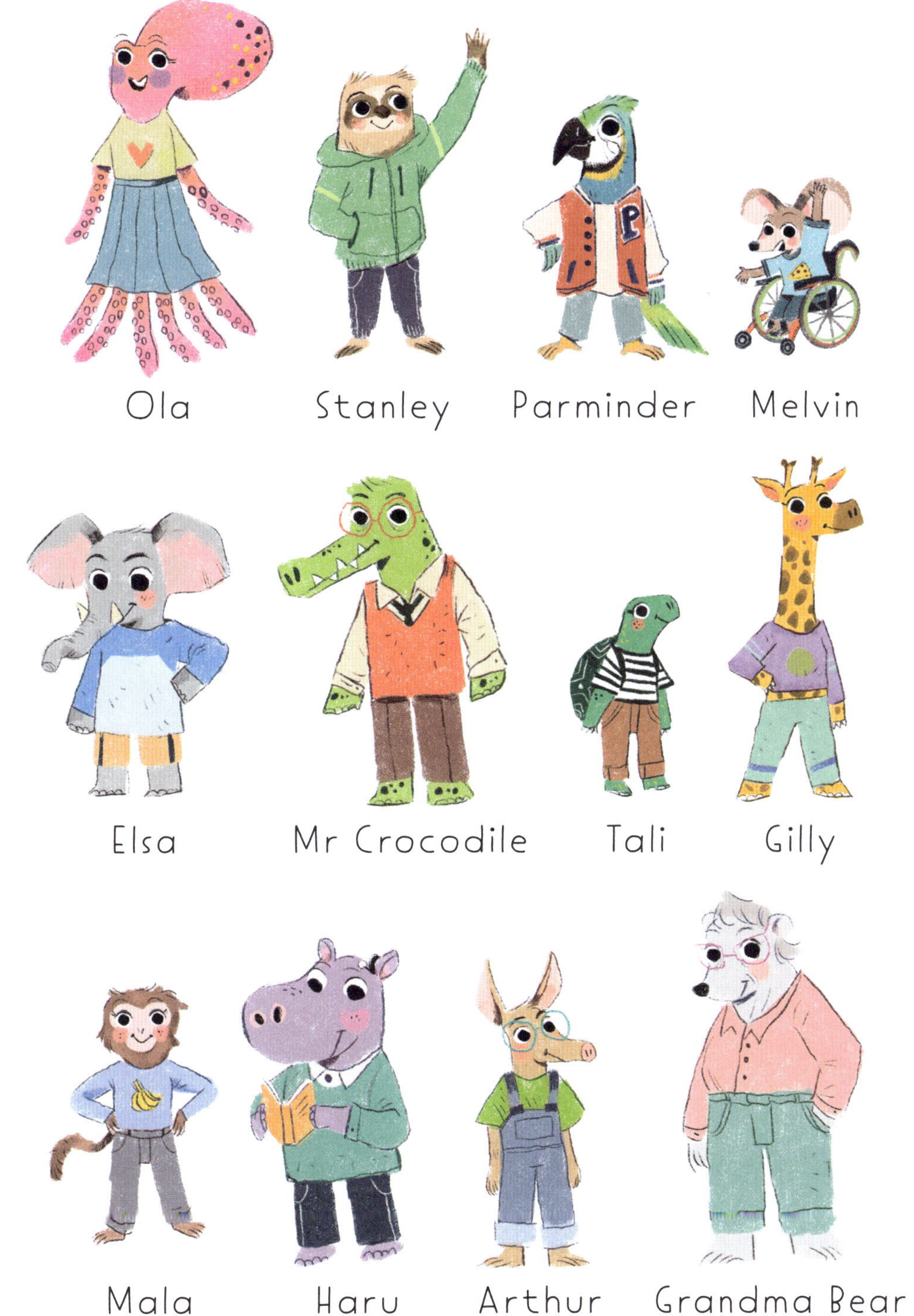

Ola Stanley Parminder Melvin

Elsa Mr Crocodile Tali Gilly

Mala Haru Arthur Grandma Bear

Talking about feelings

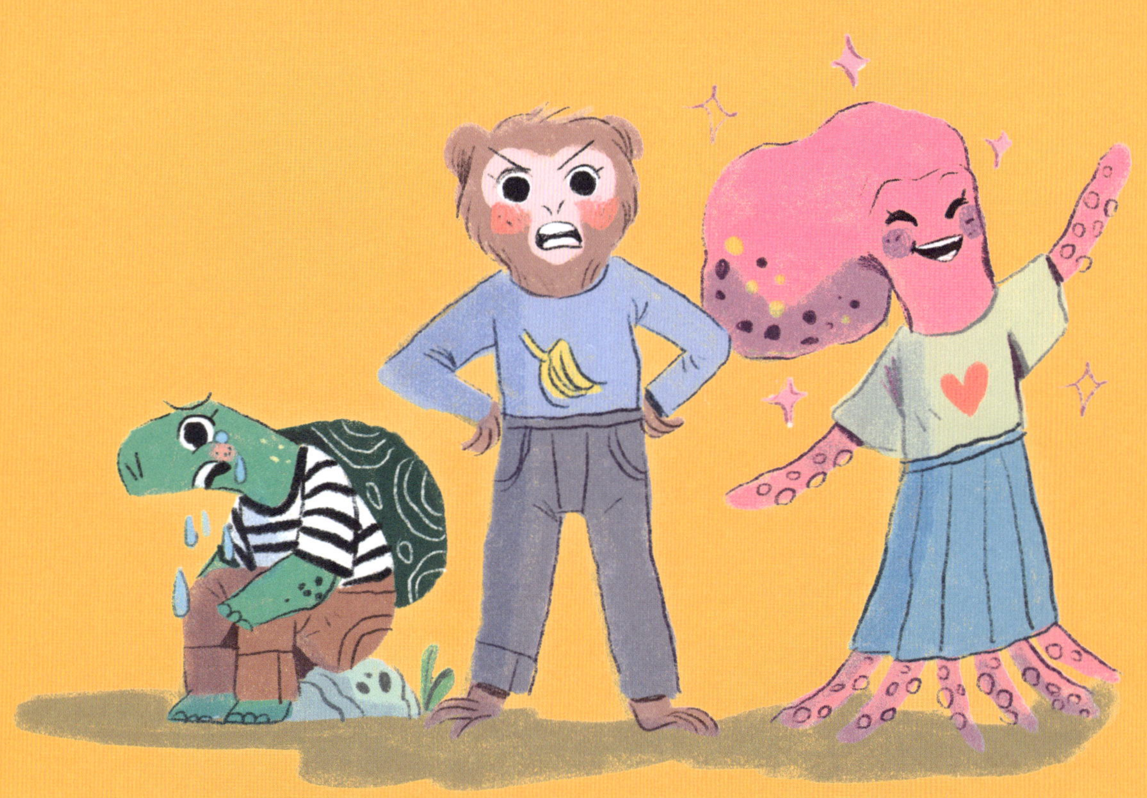

Sometimes it can be hard to know exactly how you feel. You might be grumpy or feel worried but don't know why, and that can be confusing.

Talking about feelings makes them easier to understand.

Scientists have found that when you say how you feel and talk over why you feel that way, it helps you to feel calmer. It also makes it much easier for other people to help you.

Let's practise talking about feelings.

The feelings game

Let's play the feelings game and have a go at talking about lots of different feelings.

1. Write feeling words on little pieces of paper, fold them up and pop them into a jar.
2. One person takes a piece of paper from the jar and reads it out loud.

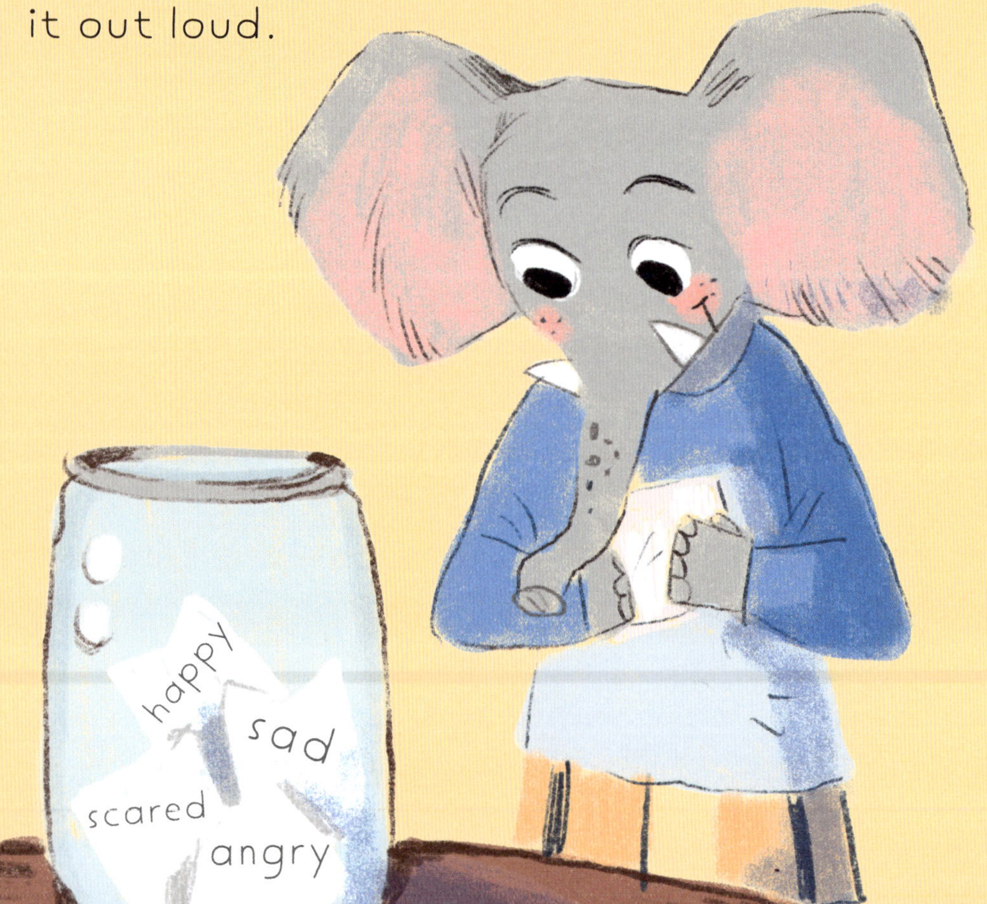

3. Starting with the picker, everyone takes a turn saying what makes them feel like the word on the paper. If someone finds it difficult, they can skip their go or ask for help.

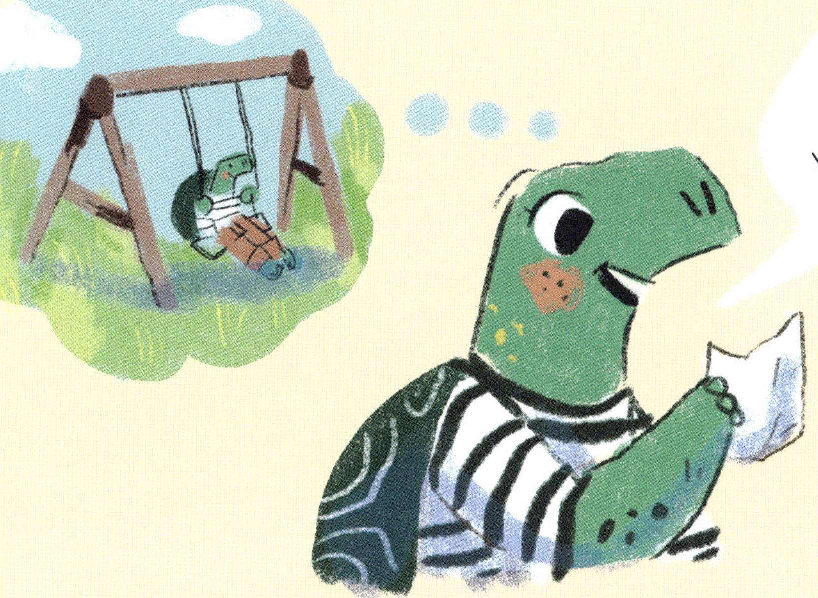

4. Then it's the next person's turn to choose from the jar. Keep going until everyone has picked a piece of paper.

The winner is – everyone who has a go!

With practice, talking about feelings gets easier and more comfortable.

For grown-ups

Children need to feel safe when being open about their feelings, so this game is best played in a small group or one-on-one with a trusted adult.

Musical moods

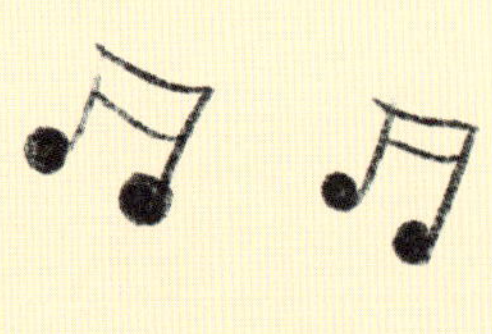

Listening to music can change how you feel. Lively music might make you want to smile and dance. Relaxing music might help you feel calm and sleepy.

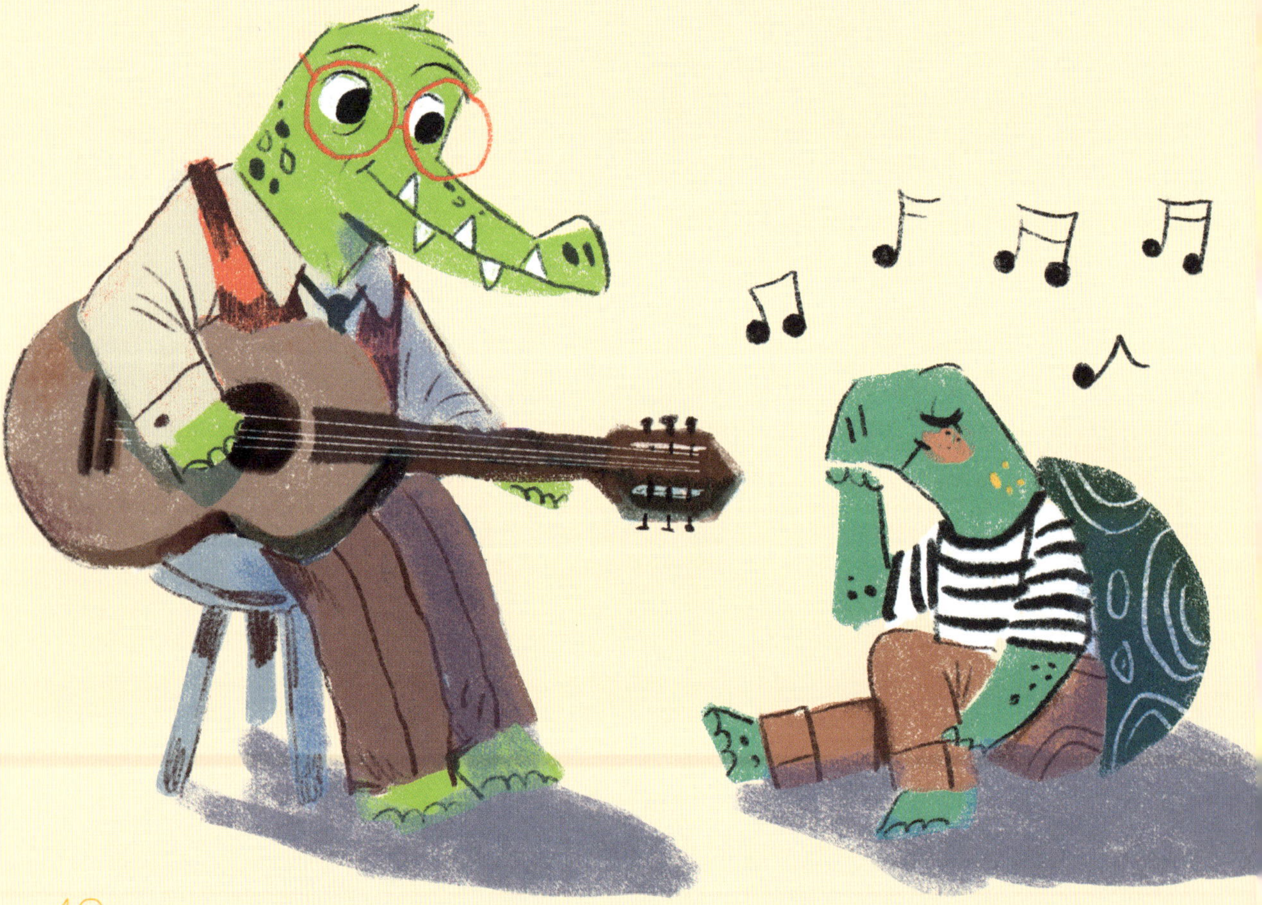

Have a listen to all these different types of music one at a time.

Hip Hop

Jazz

Rock

Pop

Classical

Say how you feel after listening to each one.

Did everyone who listened feel the same?

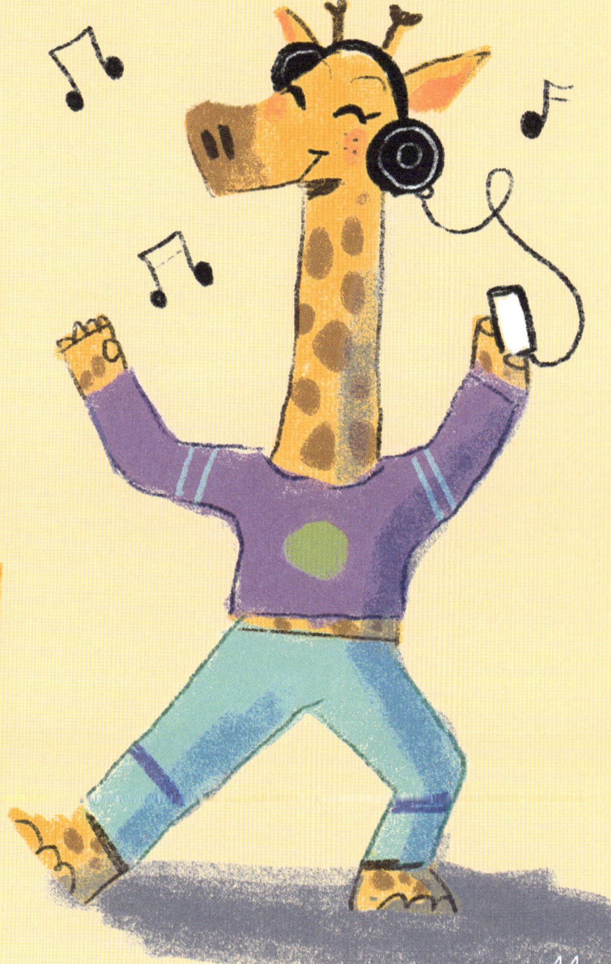

For grown-ups

Help your child create a calm-down or cheer-up playlist so they can change how they feel whenever they want.

Animal charades

Your body gives you lots of clues about how you feel. When your heart beats fast it may show you are excited, and when your face gets hot you might feel shy. When you tremble, it could be because you feel scared.

Listening to your body is useful because it helps you to understand how you feel.

Let's see how feelings show up in our bodies by playing this guessing game.

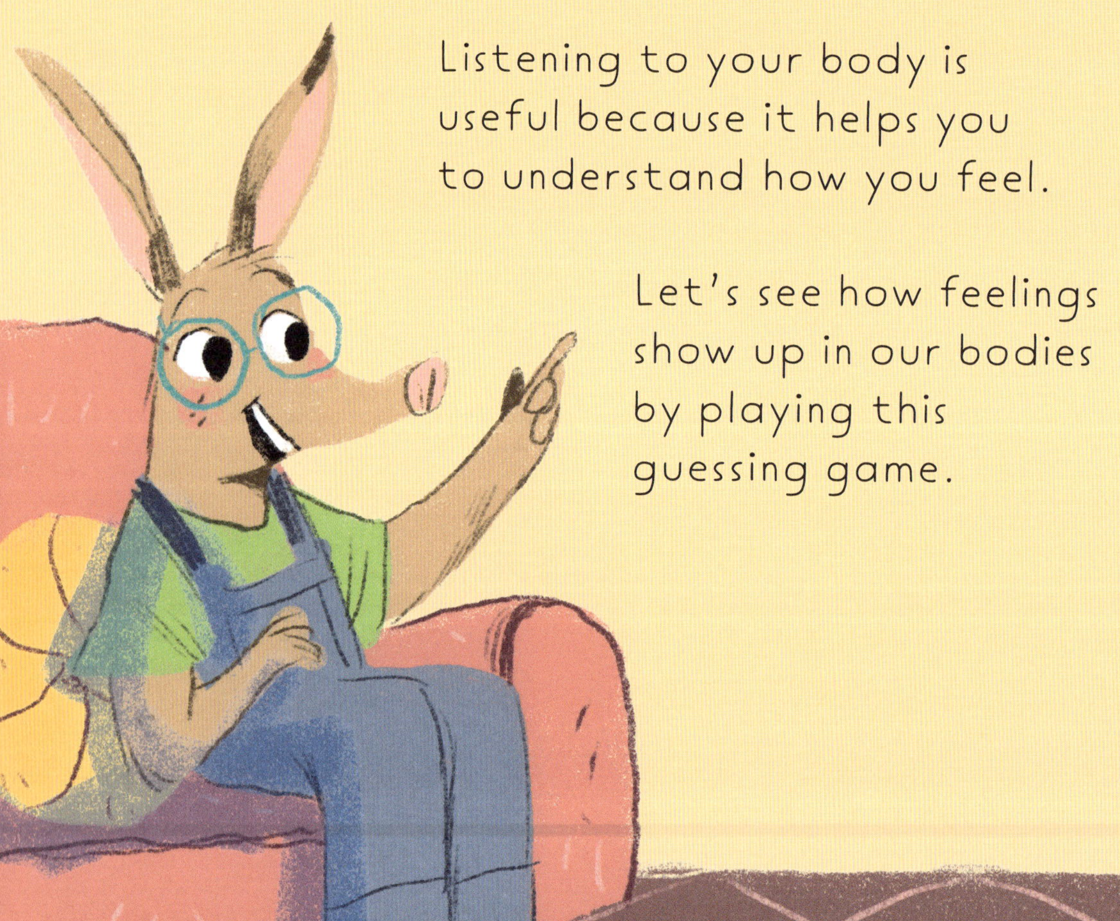

Act out the following animals (you can use sounds but not words) and see if your friends or family can guess what you are feeling and who you are.

Excited Elephant
Grumpy Giraffe
Angry Ant
Miserable Mouse
Shy Sheep
Happy Horse
Scared Snake

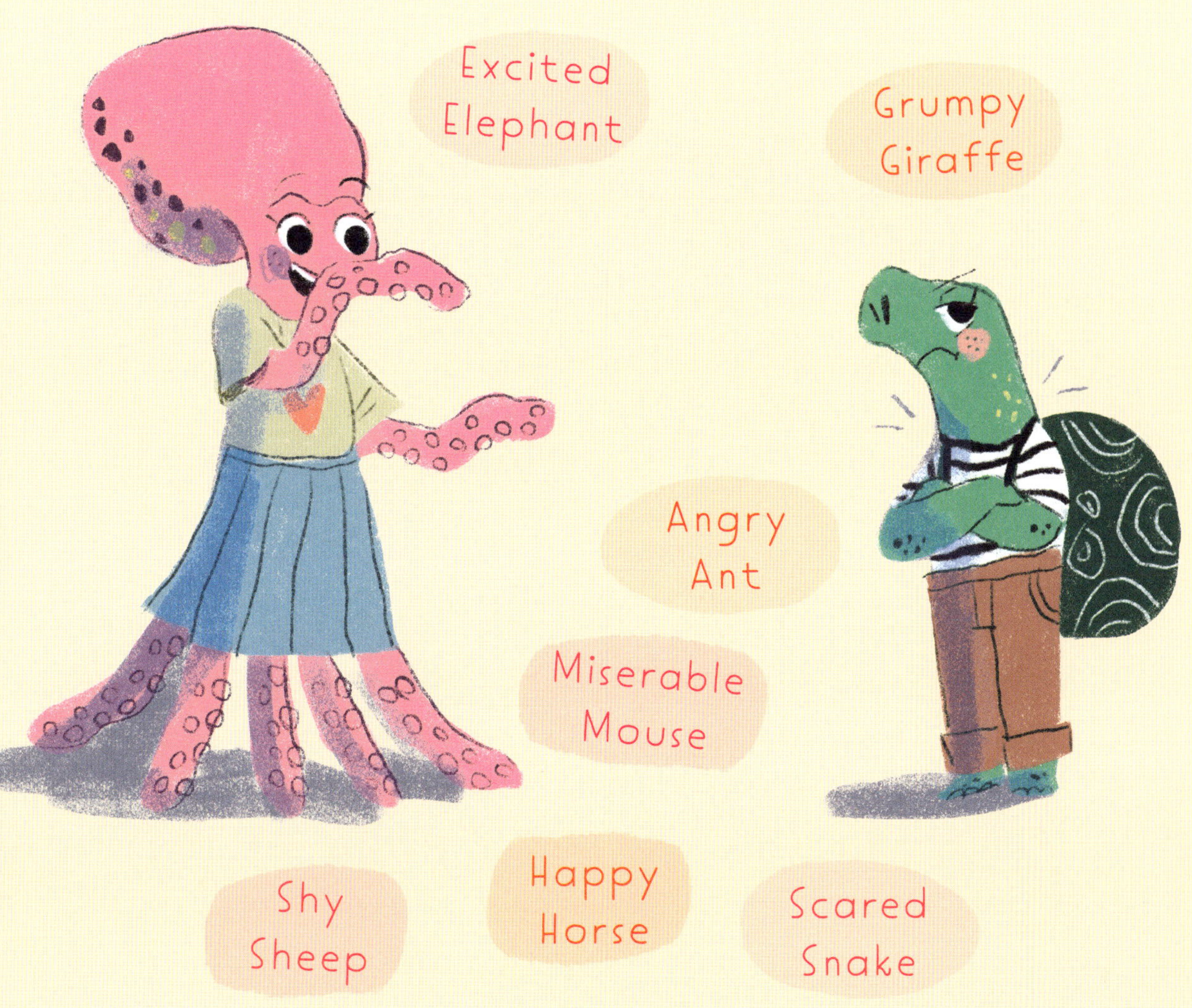

Did your friends and family find some of these hard to guess? They probably did and this is why it helps to tell people how you feel, not just expect them to guess.

A day full of feelings

Feelings come and feelings go.

Even big feelings don't last forever, and it helps to remember this when you feel upset. You don't have to fight your feelings or pretend you don't have them.

To see how your feelings change over time, make a diary on a sheet of paper, like the one on the next page. Write or draw in your feelings throughout the day.

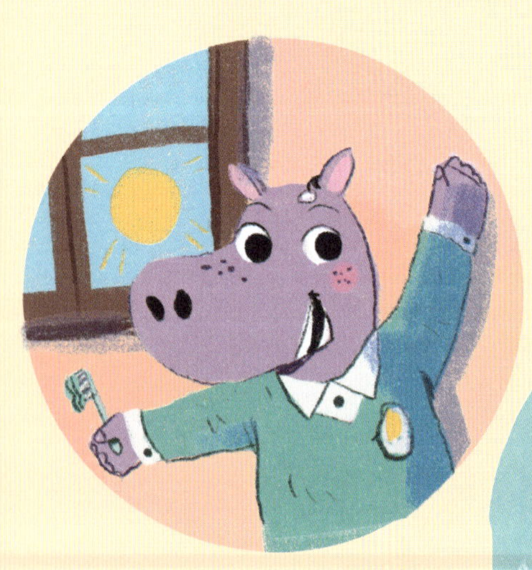

Morning

Afternoon

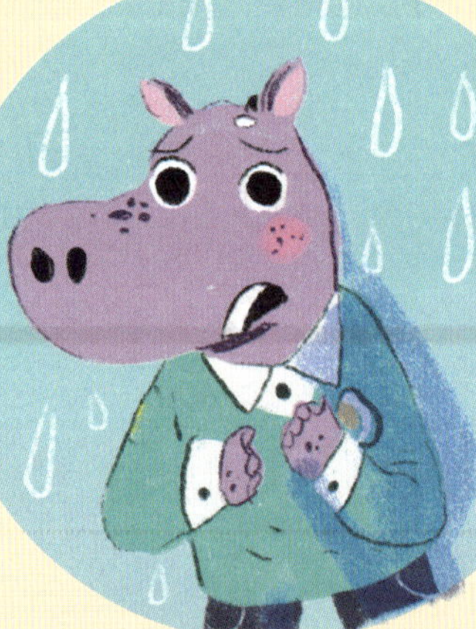

Evening

Day	Morning	Afternoon	Evening
Monday	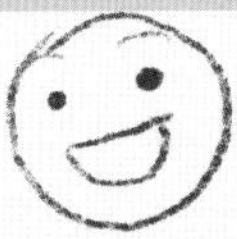	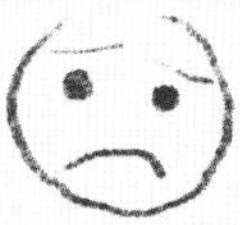	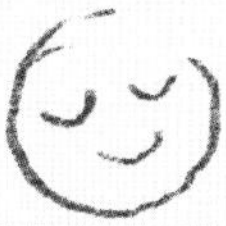
Tuesday			
Wednesday			
Thursday			
Friday			
Saturday			
Sunday			

Are you surprised how many different feelings you had in a week?

You might have more than one feeling at a time and that's totally normal. Try to name them all.

Look for clues

When you try to imagine how someone else feels it is called having empathy (em-pa-thee). Understanding how someone else feels can help you to be kinder to them and more helpful.

What do you think these animals are feeling? Look at their bodies and faces for clues and think about what has happened to them.

Haru Hippo can't tie his shoelaces.

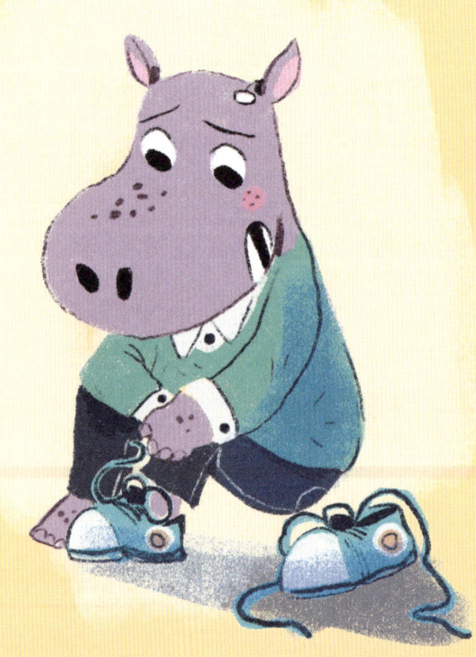

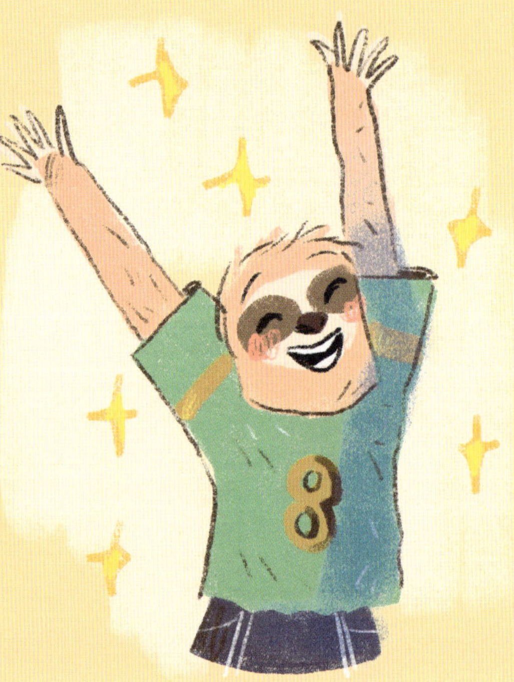

Stanley Sloth just scored a goal.

Tali Turtle
broke her toy.

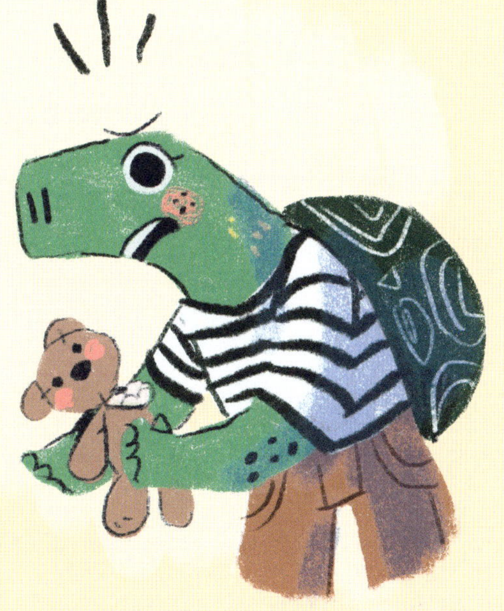

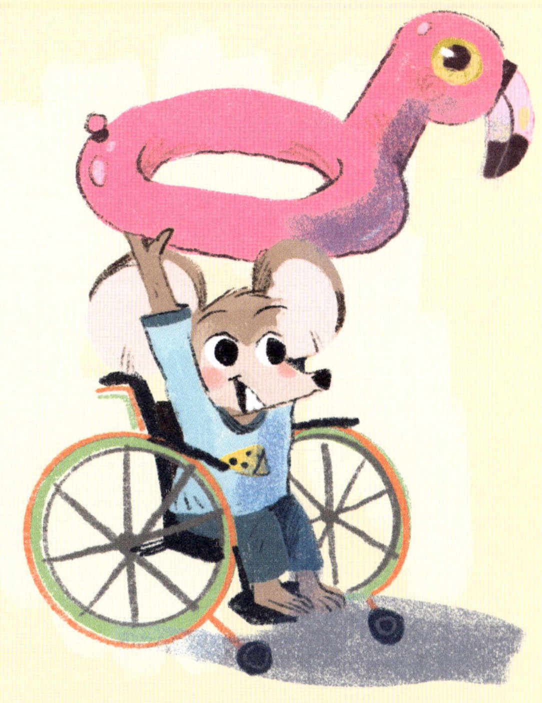

Melvin Mouse is
going on holiday.

Elsa Elephant is
moving house.

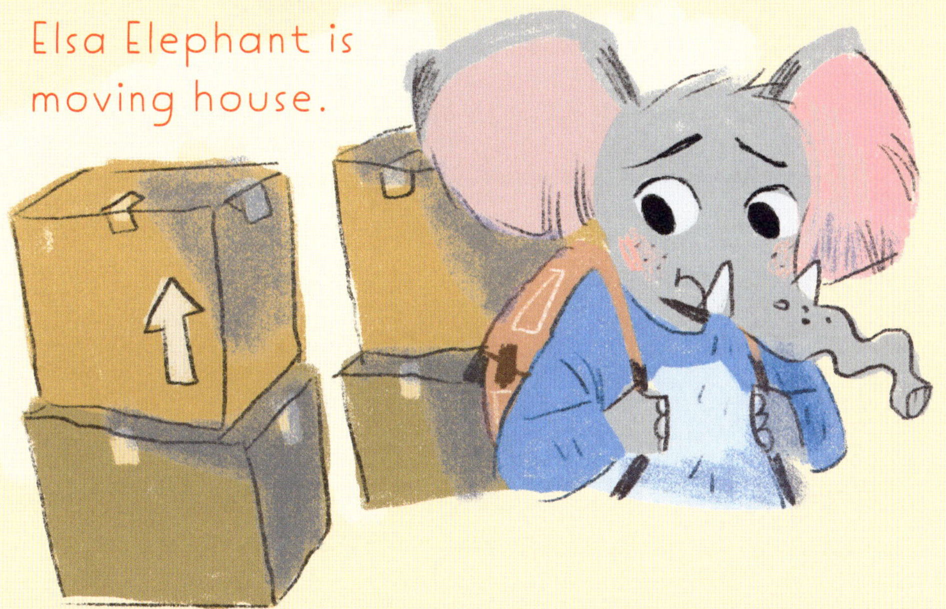

If you aren't sure how somebody feels, you can always ask them 'How do you feel?' and they will probably tell you.

The feelings alphabet

There are hundreds of amazing feeling words.

The more words you have to describe how you feel the better. It will help you and other people understand your emotions and how to help you.

Have a go at drawing the first letter of your name as a feeling word. Maybe you would like to write your whole name this way.

For grown-ups

Some of the feelings on the next page might need putting into sentences to help a child understand their meaning. Drawing your own feelings alphabet alongside your child is a great opportunity to chat more about emotions.

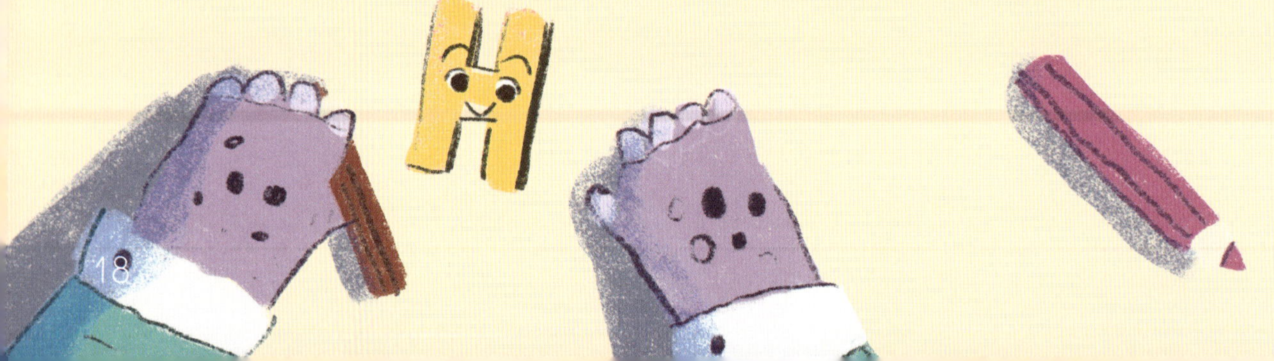

Here are some examples of feelings for each letter of the alphabet.

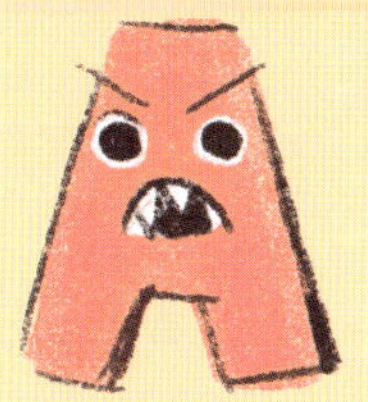
Angry

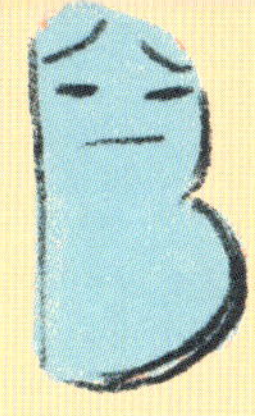
Bored

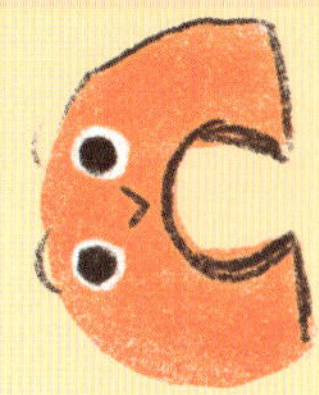
Calm

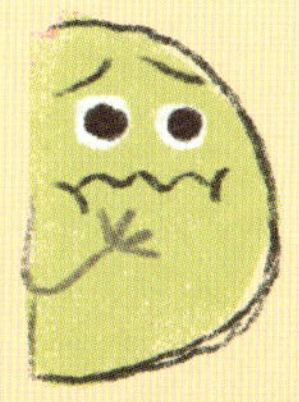
Disgusted

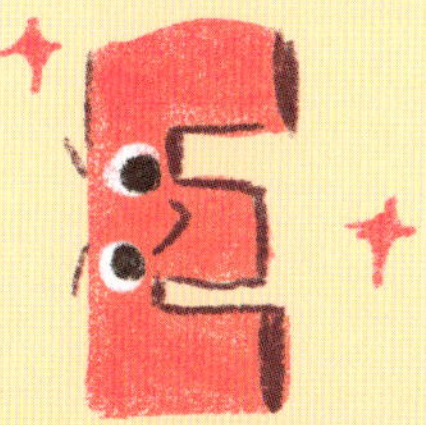
Energetic

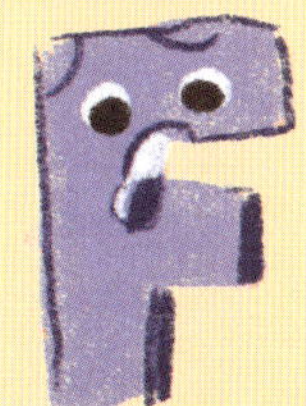
Frightened

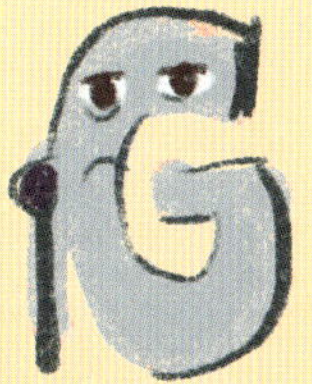
Grumpy

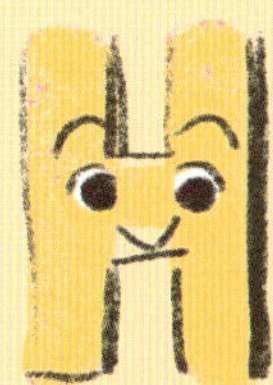
Happy

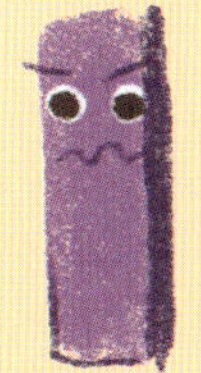
Irritated

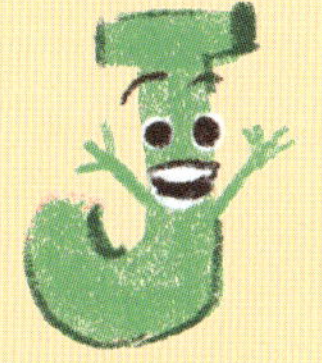
Joyful

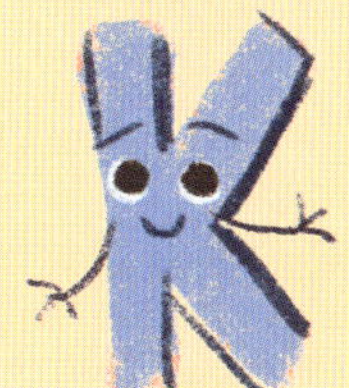
Kind

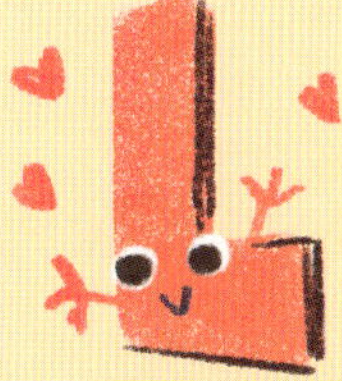
Loving

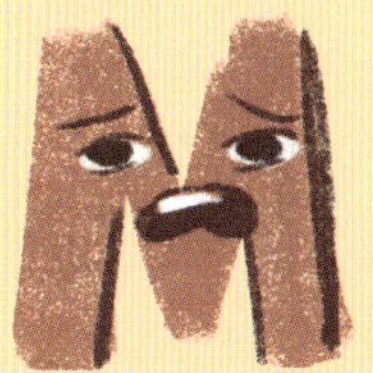
Miserable

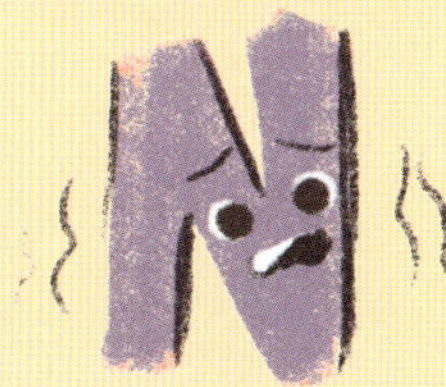
Nervous

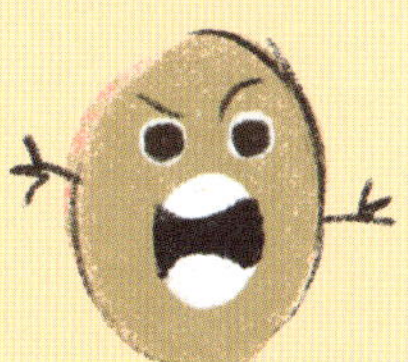
Outraged

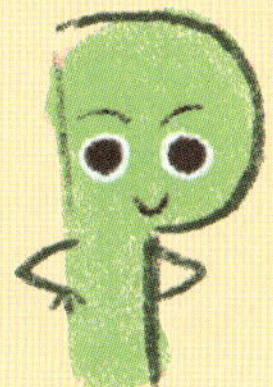
Proud

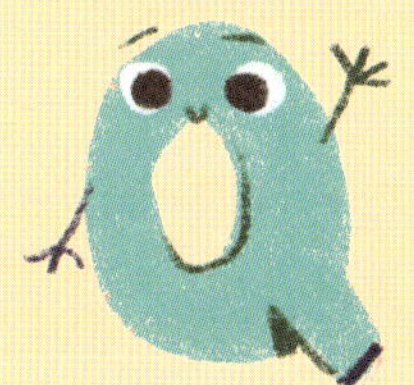
Questioning

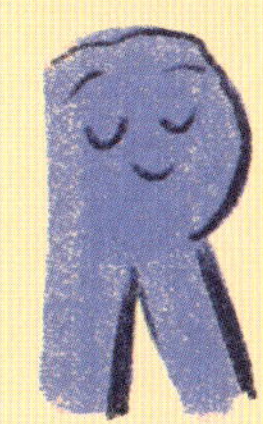
Restful

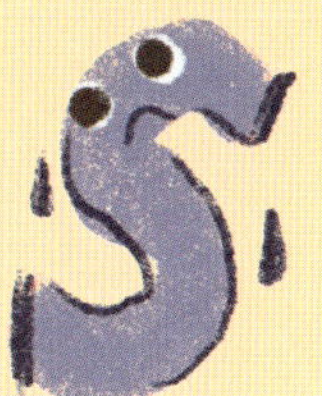
Sad

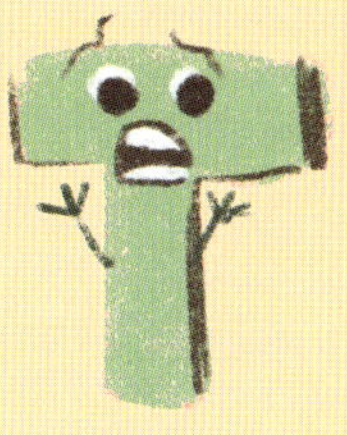
Terrified

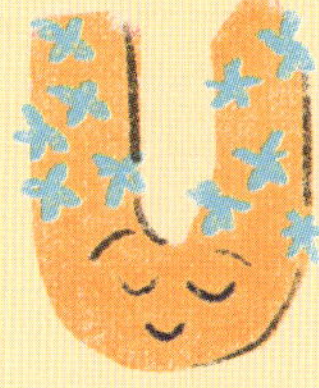
Unique

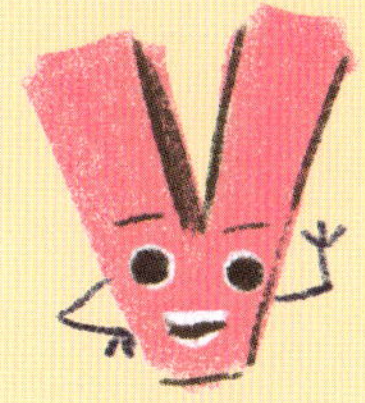
Valued

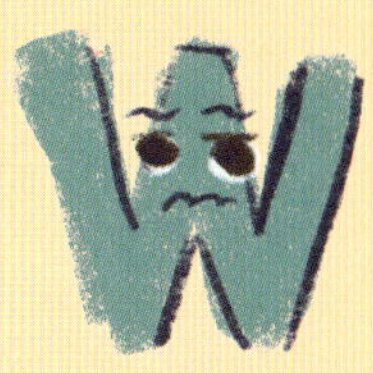
Worried

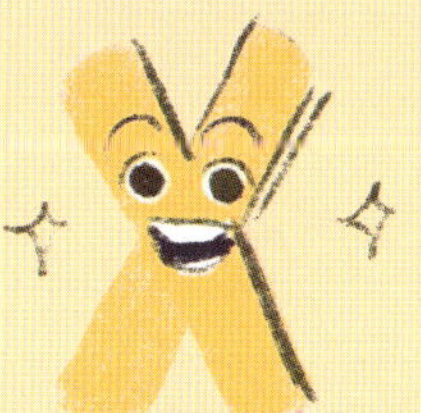
eXcited

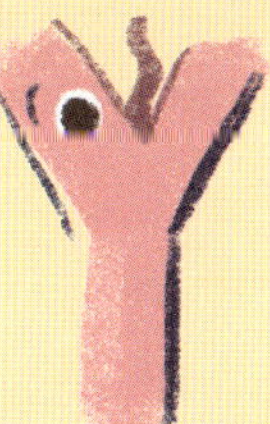
Yucky

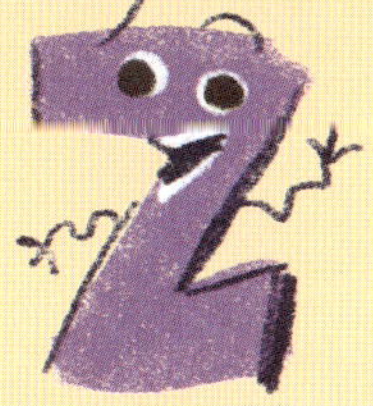
Zany

Show your feelings

People often show their feelings in the way they behave. You know lots of feeling words now, so have a go at finishing these sentences ....

I cry when I feel ...

I stamp when I feel ...

I shout when I feel ...

I go quiet when I feel ...

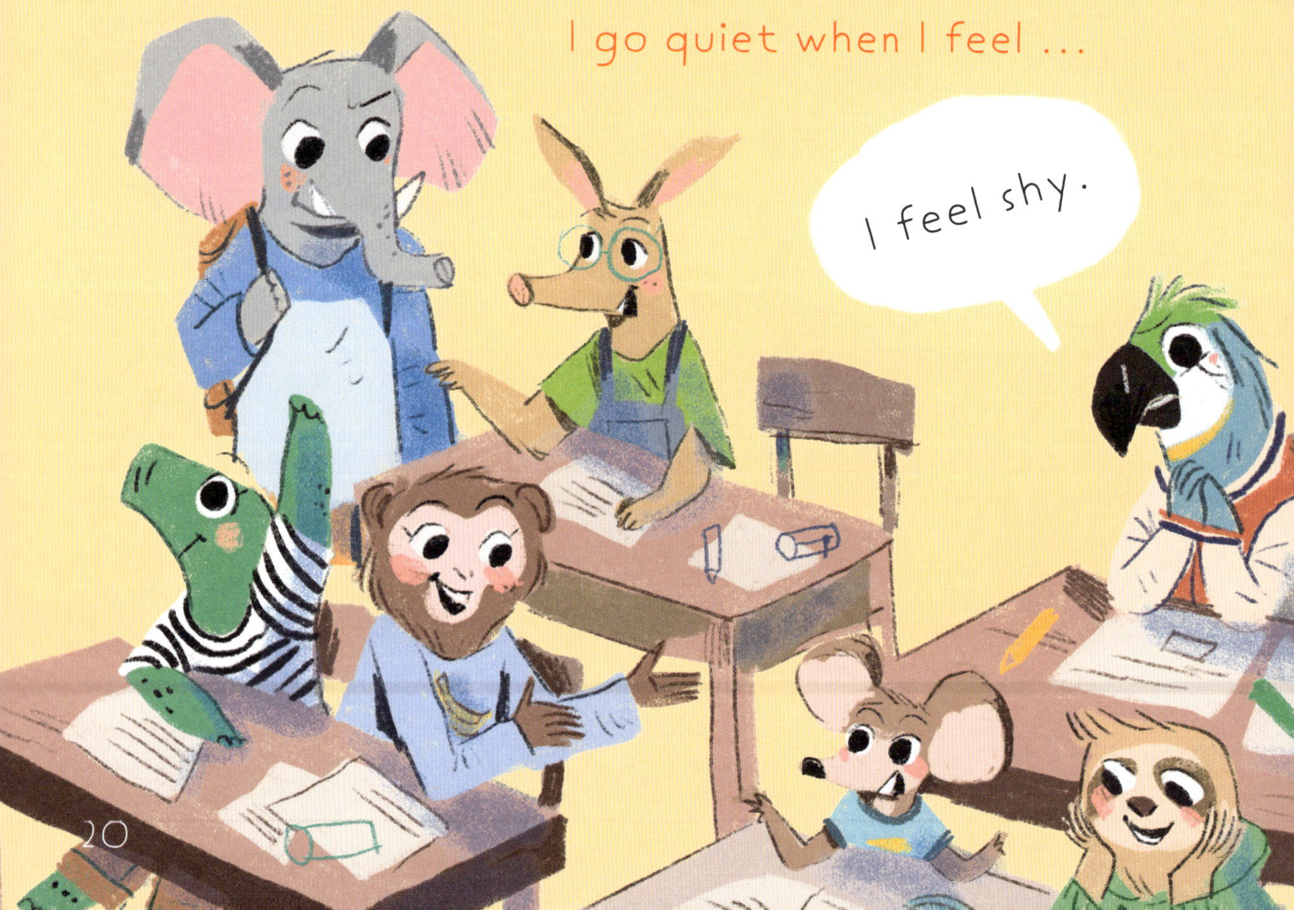

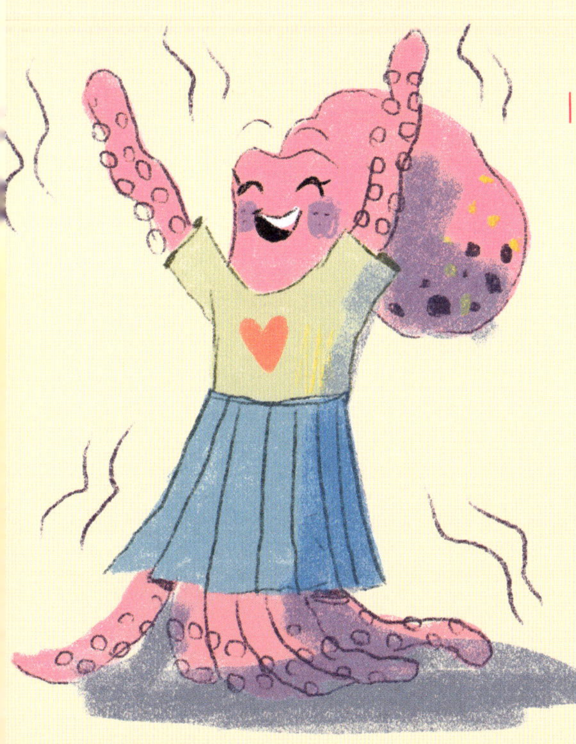

I dance when I feel ...

I laugh when I feel ...

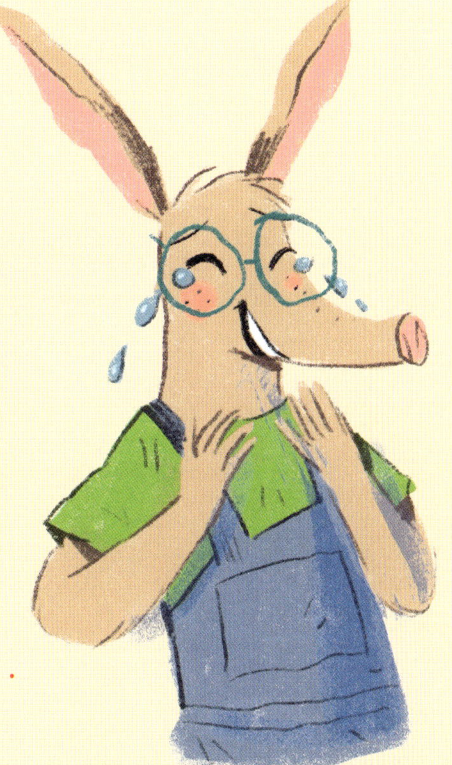

I jump about when I feel ...

I shiver when I feel ...

Not everyone shows their feelings in the same way. People may not understand what you are showing them with just your actions. This is why using words for your feelings can be really helpful.

For grown-ups

Complete this exercise alongside your child to demonstrate how people express feelings differently.

Let your feelings out

Words are brilliant but there are other fun and creative ways to show how you feel and stop your feelings getting bottled up inside. Letting your emotions out can feel amazing!

Paint a picture of something that scares you.
Angrily beat on a drum.
Write a happy or sad story about how you feel.

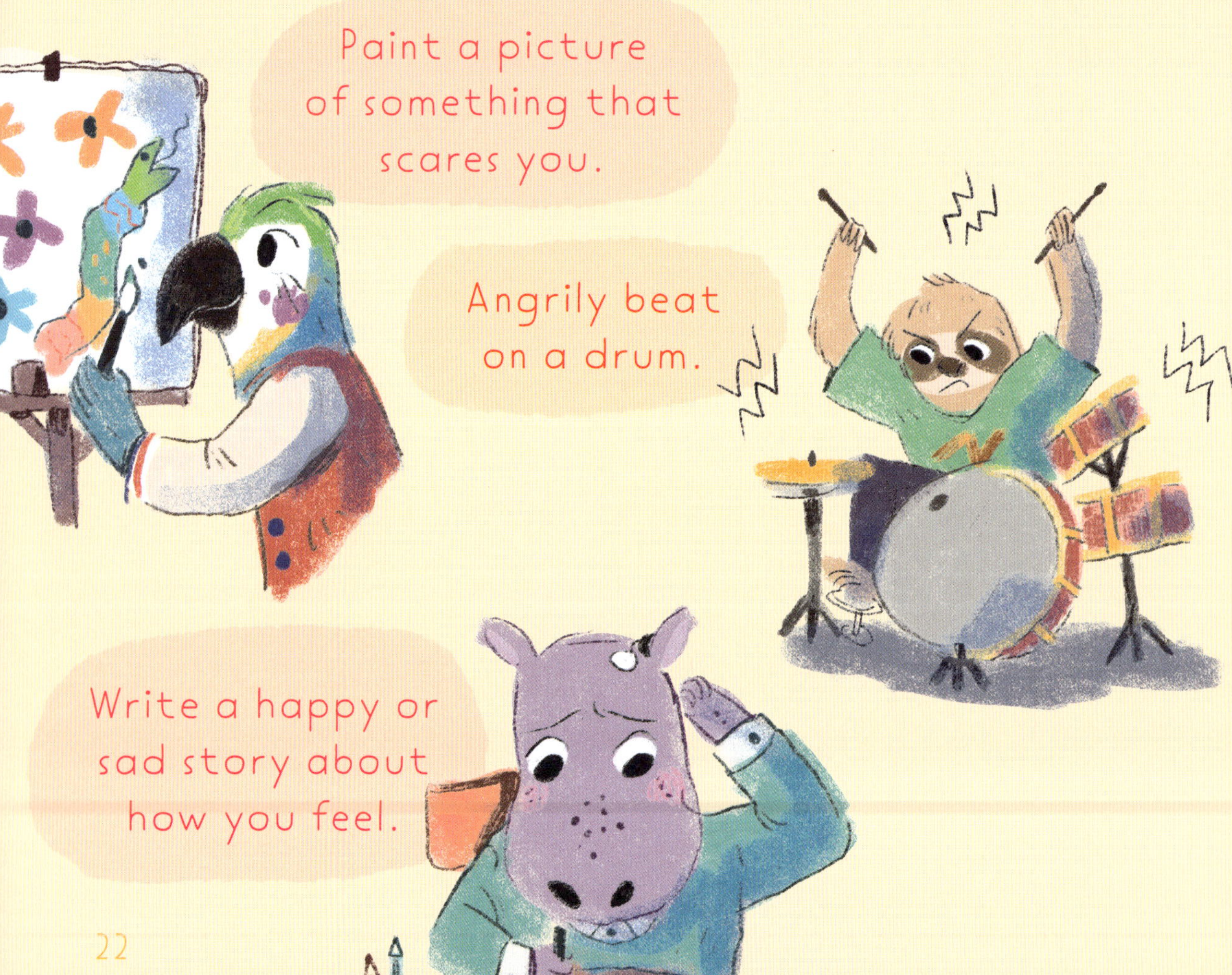

What can you make or do today to let your feelings out?

You could pick one of the ways shown here or think of something yourself?

Build a big tower then knock it down because you are annoyed.
Do a dance to show you are excited.
Laaaa
La
La
La
Sing a cheerful song.

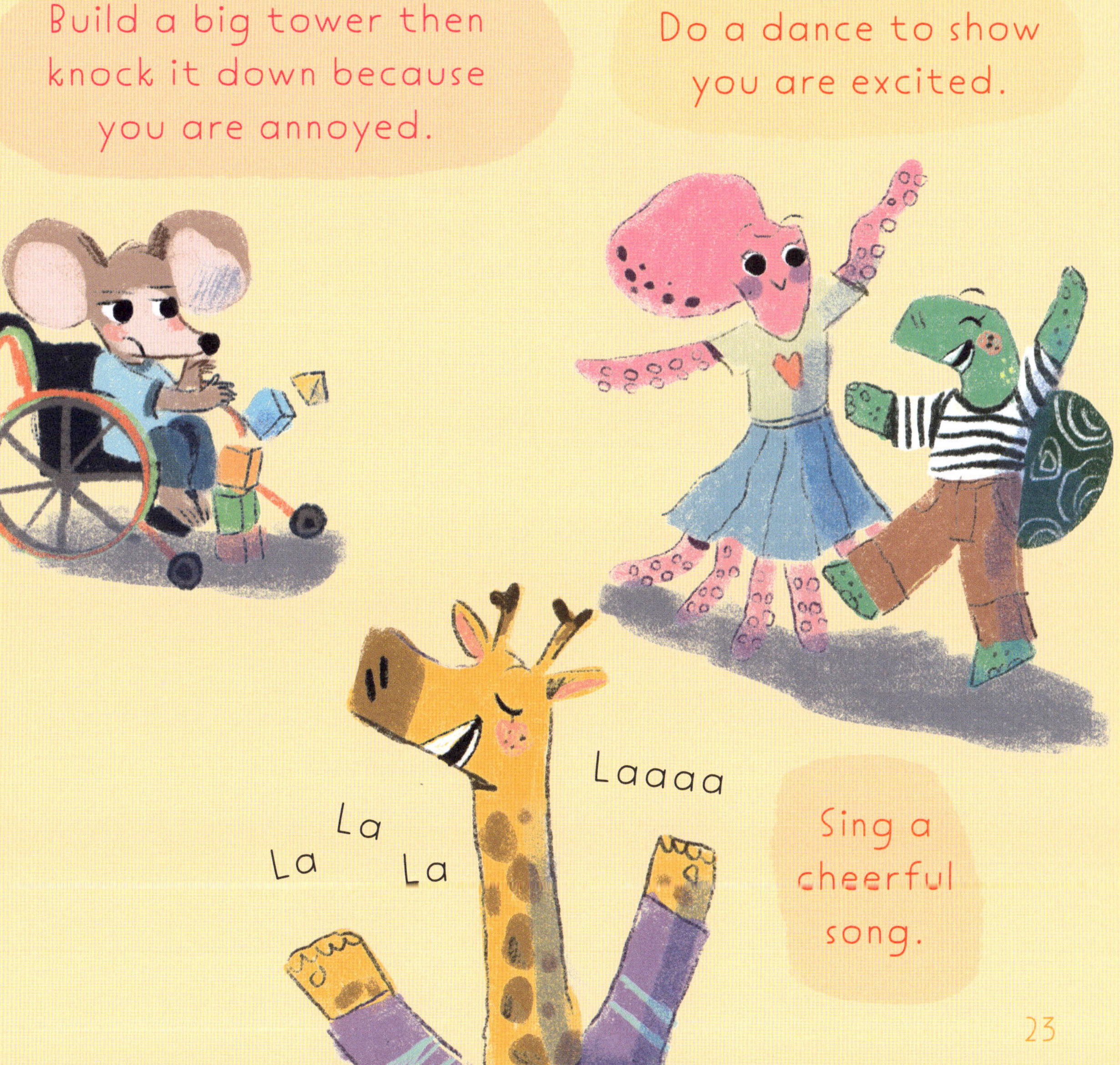

Happier

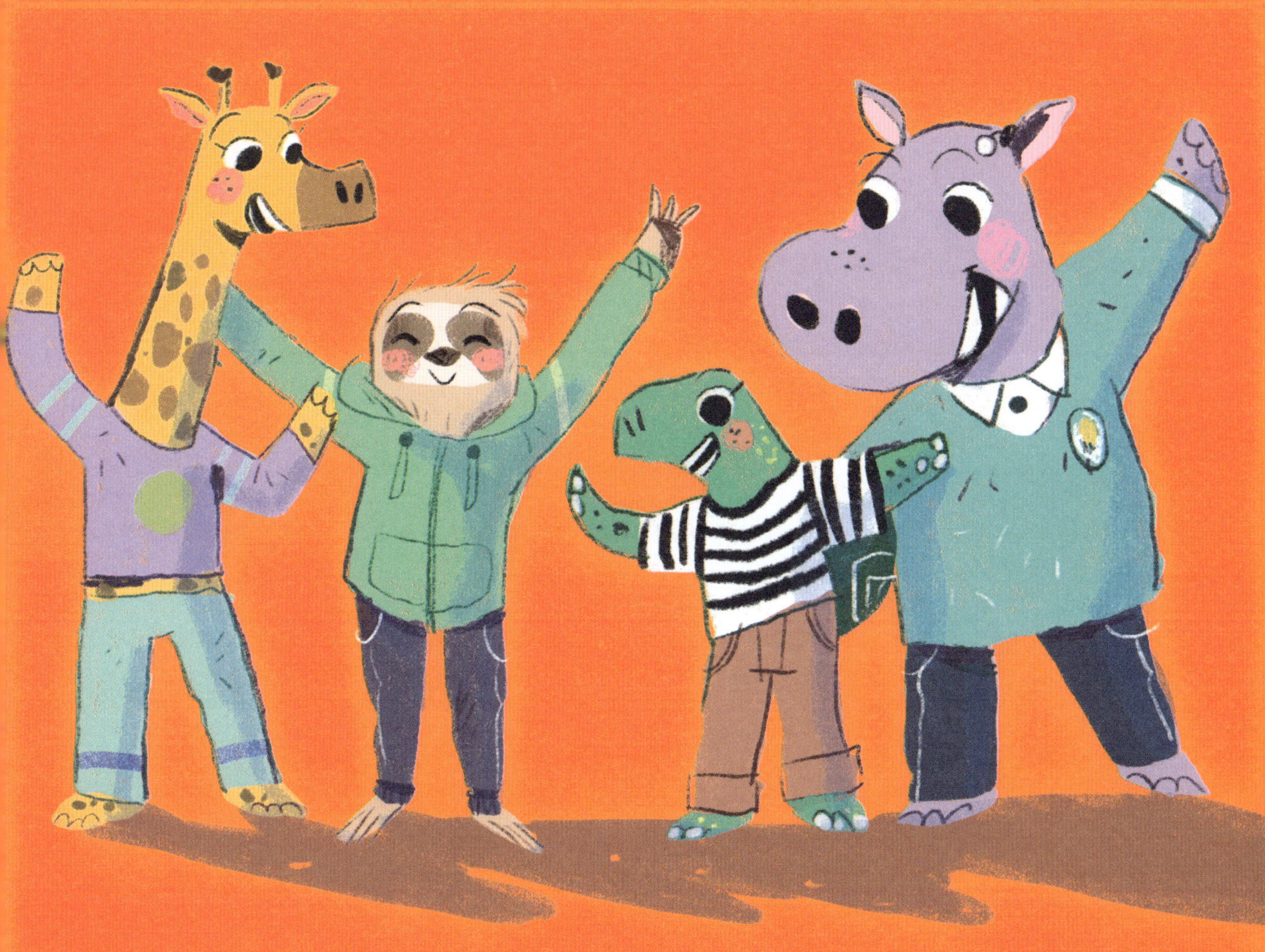

You have the power to make yourself feel happy.

Talking and thinking about things that make you smile will make you feel happier. Doing fun things that you enjoy will make you feel happier too.

There are lots of great ways to cheer yourself up.

Let's take a look.

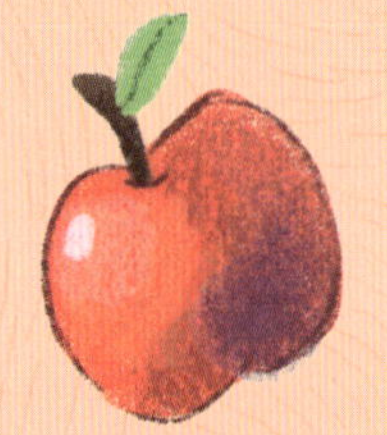

Make a happy list

If you think about things that make you happy you will feel happier.

So, let's have a go at making a happy list filled with all the things that make you smile. You can include colours, pets, people, games, places – anything you like.

You can draw it, write it, or tell someone all about it.

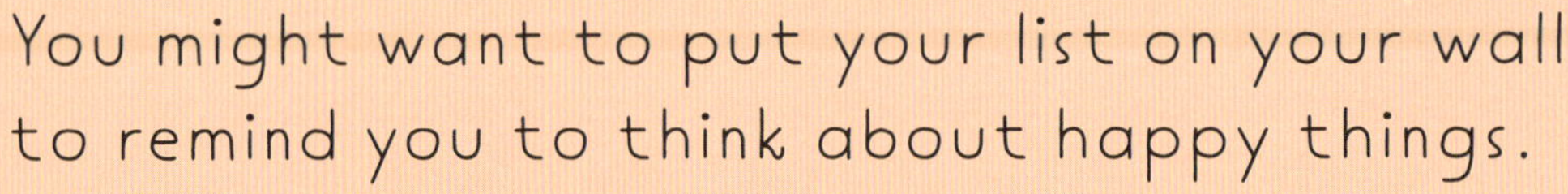

You might want to put your list on your wall to remind you to think about happy things.

H is for Hats

A is for Apples

P is for Parks

P is for Penguins

I is for Ice Cream

N is for Nice friends

E is for Elephants

S is for Seaside

S is for Smiles

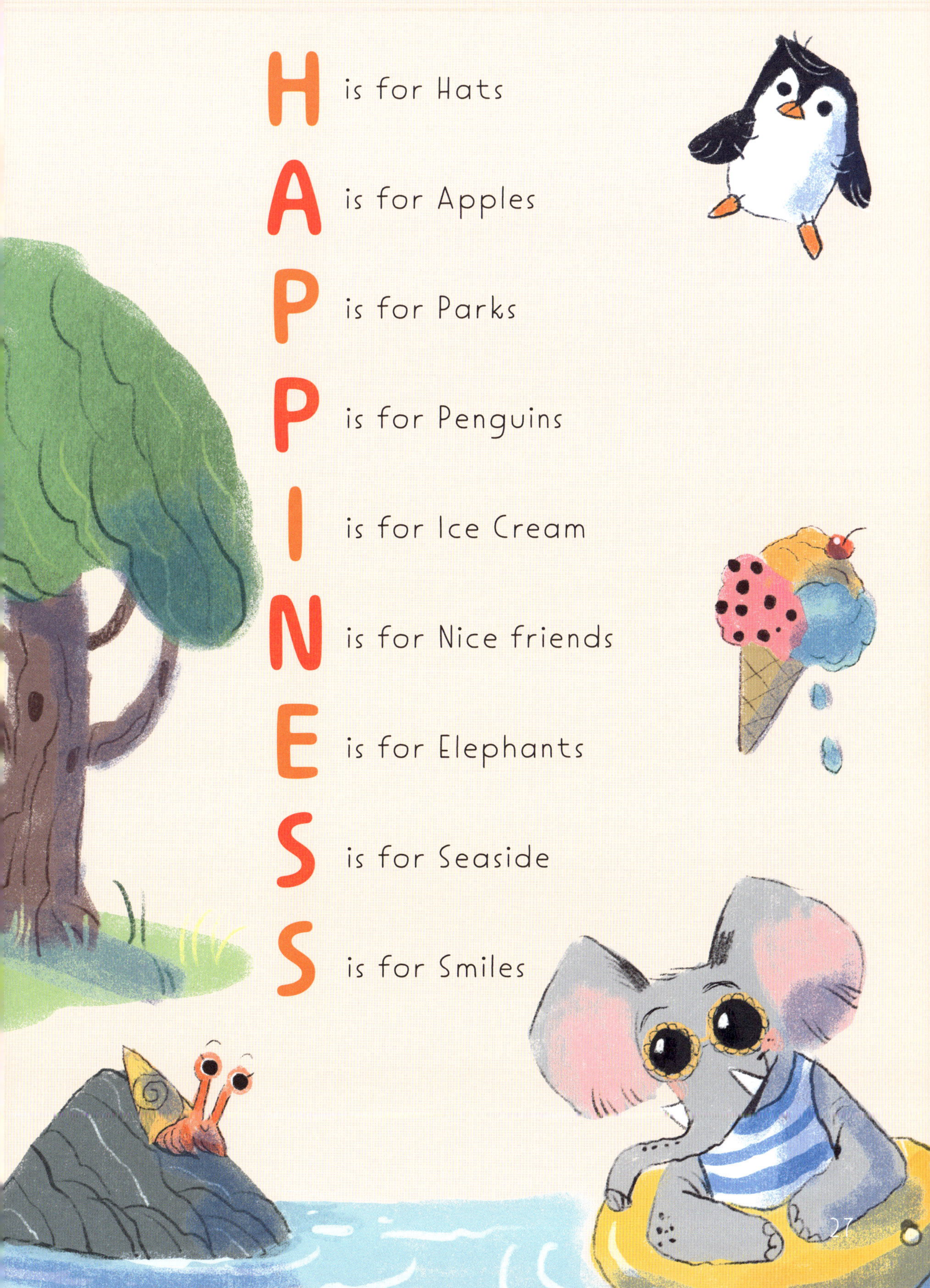

Go on a happiness hunt

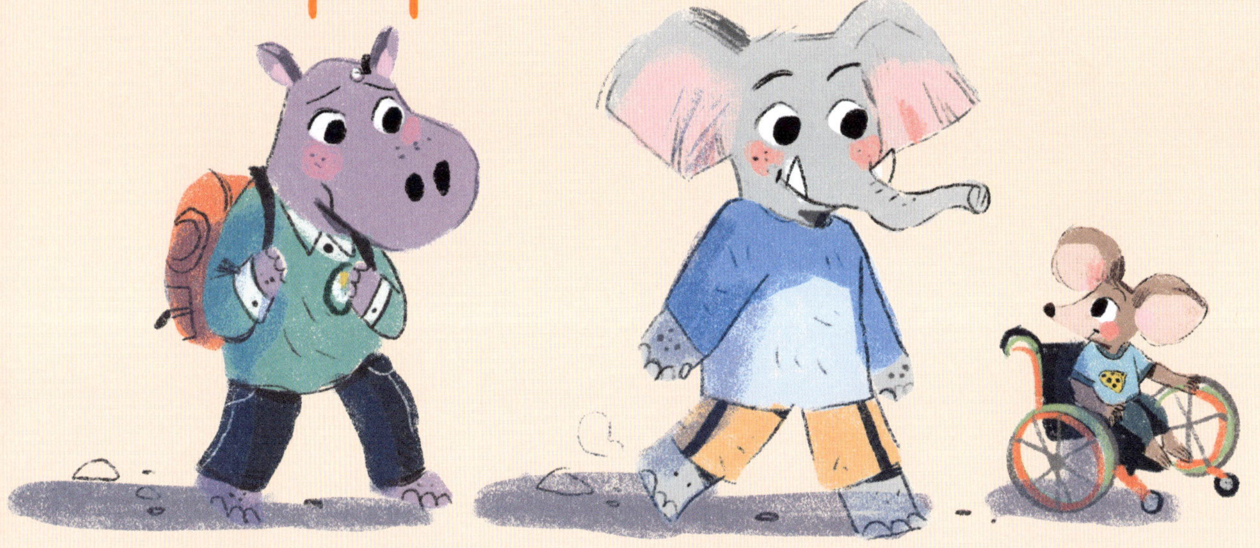

You don't have to wait for the school holidays or for your birthday for life to be amazing and for you to be happy. Lots of simple, everyday things are great too. They are easy to miss though if you don't look out for them.

So, let's go happiness hunting!

Find 10 everyday things in your house or garden that make you happy. When you find something that makes you happy, say a little thank you to it.

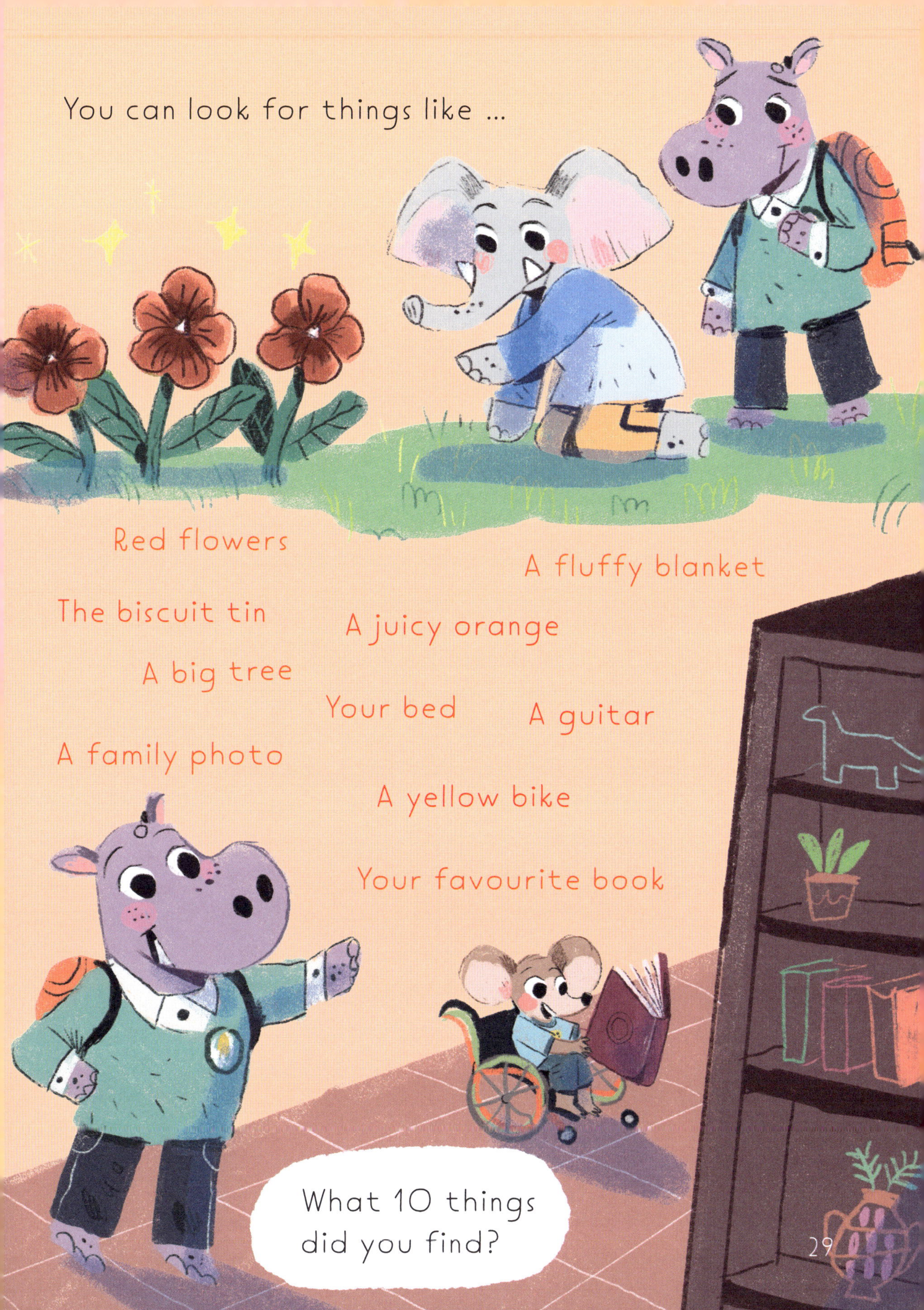

You can look for things like ...

Red flowers

A fluffy blanket

The biscuit tin

A juicy orange

A big tree

Your bed

A guitar

A family photo

A yellow bike

Your favourite book

Find your happy helpers

It is normal to feel unhappy sometimes.

When you are feeling unhappy, other people can be a big help.

Think about all the different people who could help you.

Who would ...

help you solve a problem at home?

make you laugh?

sit with you when you have a cry?

give you a hug?

listen to you talk about your feelings?

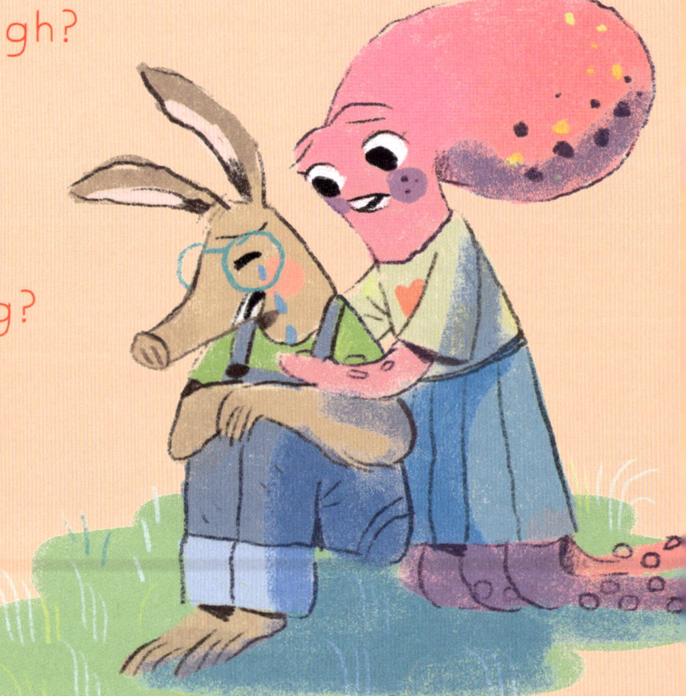

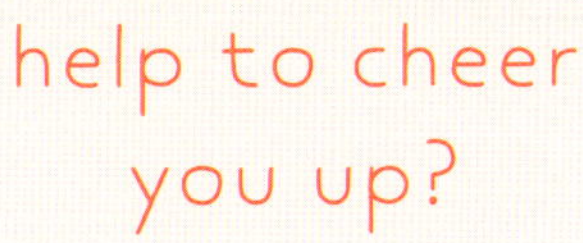

help to cheer you up?

do a fun activity with you to take your mind off things?

help you solve a problem at school?

be a good friend?

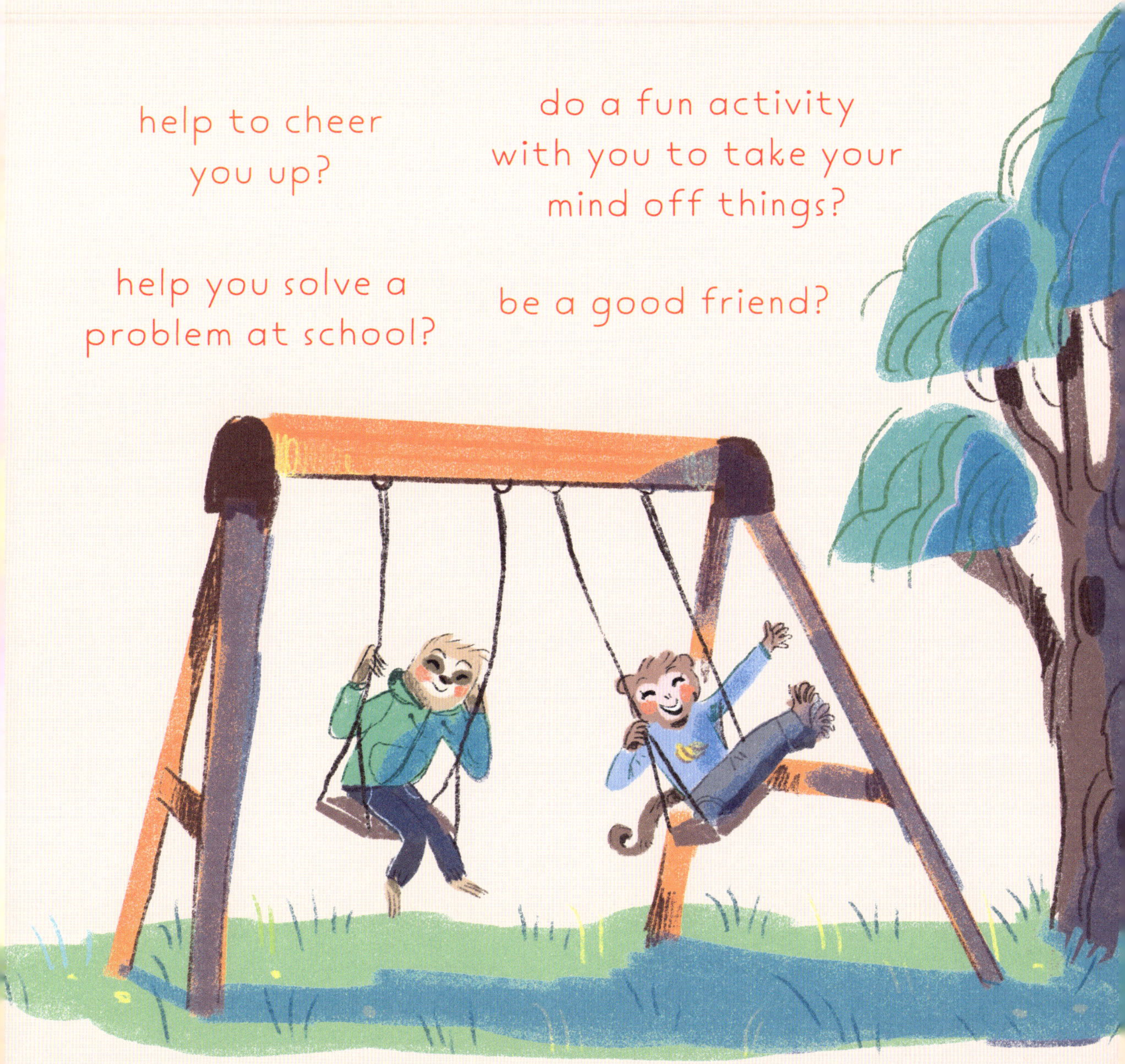

Knowing who your helpers are, and asking them to support you, can make you feel better.

You might want to write your helpers names down, so you don't forget them.

Are you a good helper?

Give a thank you card

When you say thank you to other people it makes them feel happy.

And scientists have found that when you say thank you (and really mean it) it makes you feel happy too.

Let's make a thank you card and make someone smile.

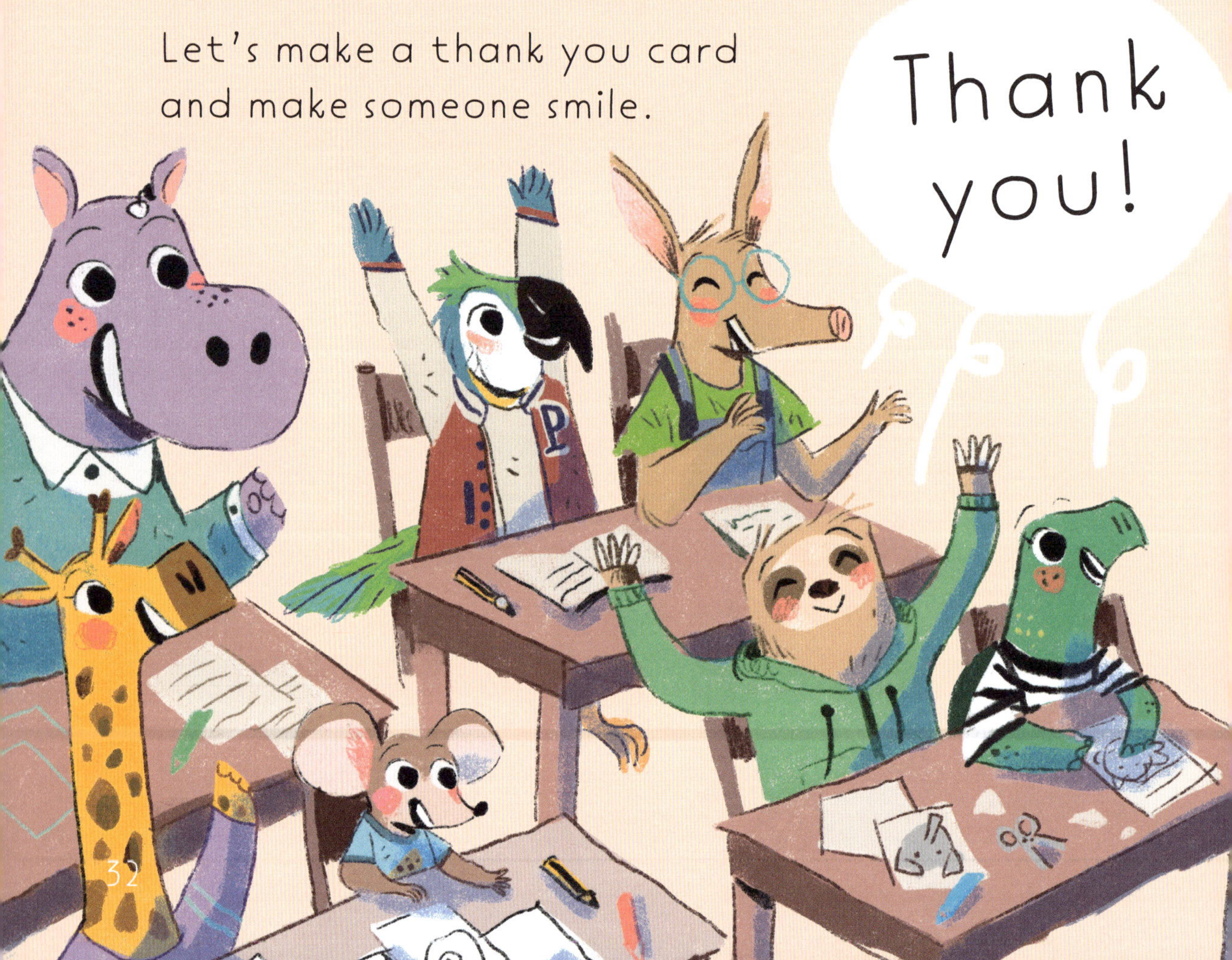

1. Think about who you could send a thank you card to – maybe your teacher, sports coach or a family member?
2. Make your card any way you want. You could use stickers, felt tips and even glue on bits of nature.
3. Say or draw what you are thanking them for.
4. Don't forget to put their name and your name on it too.
5. Now deliver your card. It will make you both smile.

If it felt good to give a thank you card you might want to make some more.

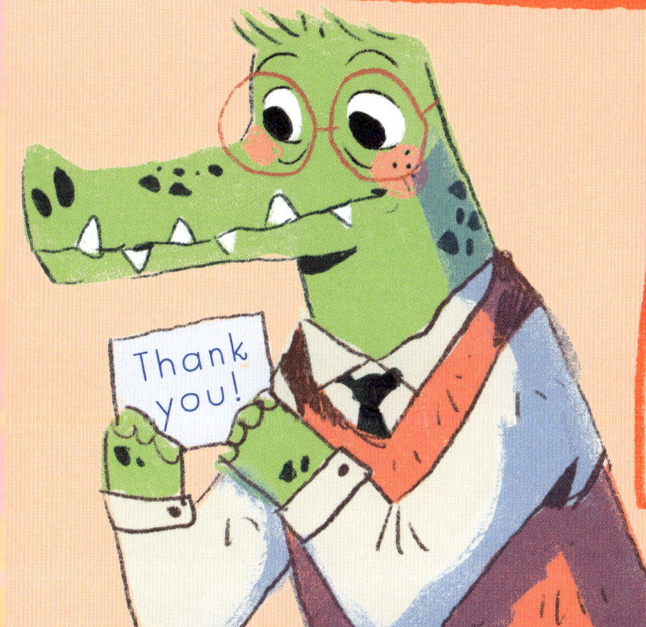

For grown-ups

Reflecting on things to be thankful for is a lovely activity to share with your child at bedtime. It enables them to fall asleep with a mind free from worries and full of warm and happy thoughts.

What went well

When something goes wrong it is easy to just think about that and forget all the things that went right.

Maybe you dropped your bag in a puddle today but you made a new friend.

Perhaps you fell over at playtime but you had your favourite pudding.

It's important to talk about what went wrong and get support if you need it, but it is also really important to remember what went well too.

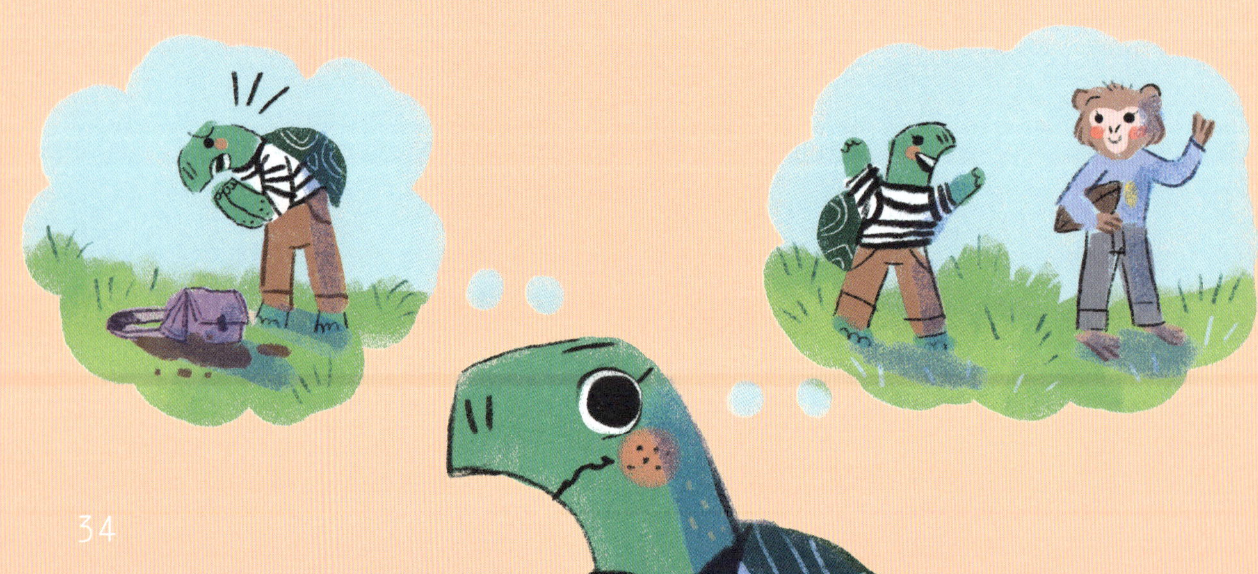

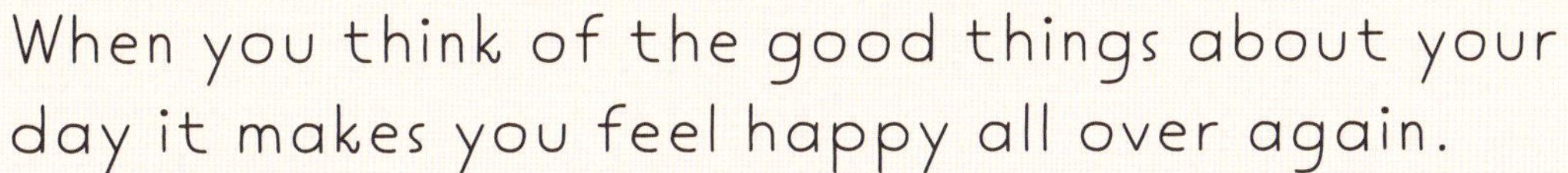

When you think of the good things about your day it makes you feel happy all over again.

Try talking about what went well for you today at tea-time or on the way home from school.

Can you think of 3 different things?

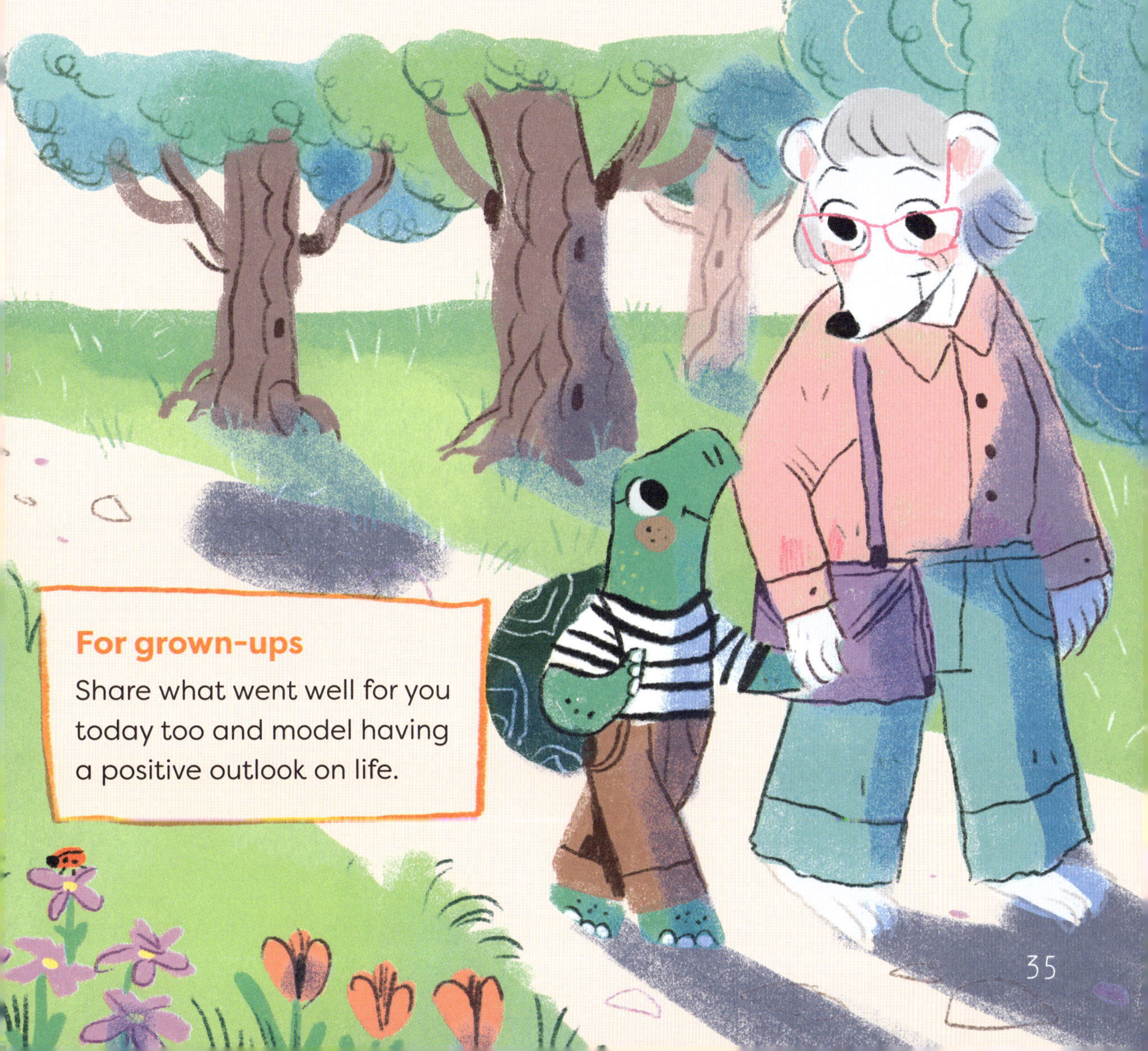

For grown-ups

Share what went well for you today too and model having a positive outlook on life.

Make a nature face

Scientists have found that spending time in nature makes you feel happy. Exercise makes you happy too, so going on a nature walk is a great idea.

Take a bag or bucket with you to collect lots of little bits of nature that have already fallen to the ground.

Be sure to wash your hands after picking them up!

Look for things like ...

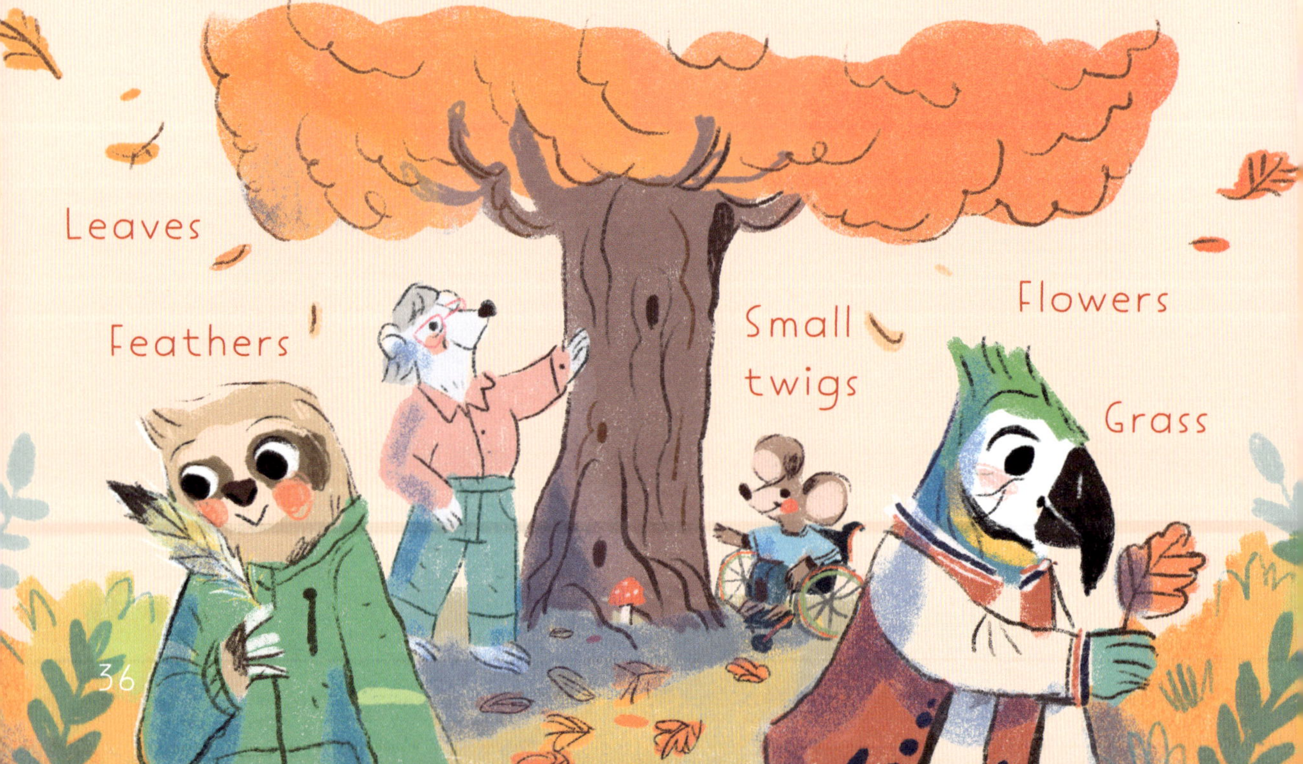

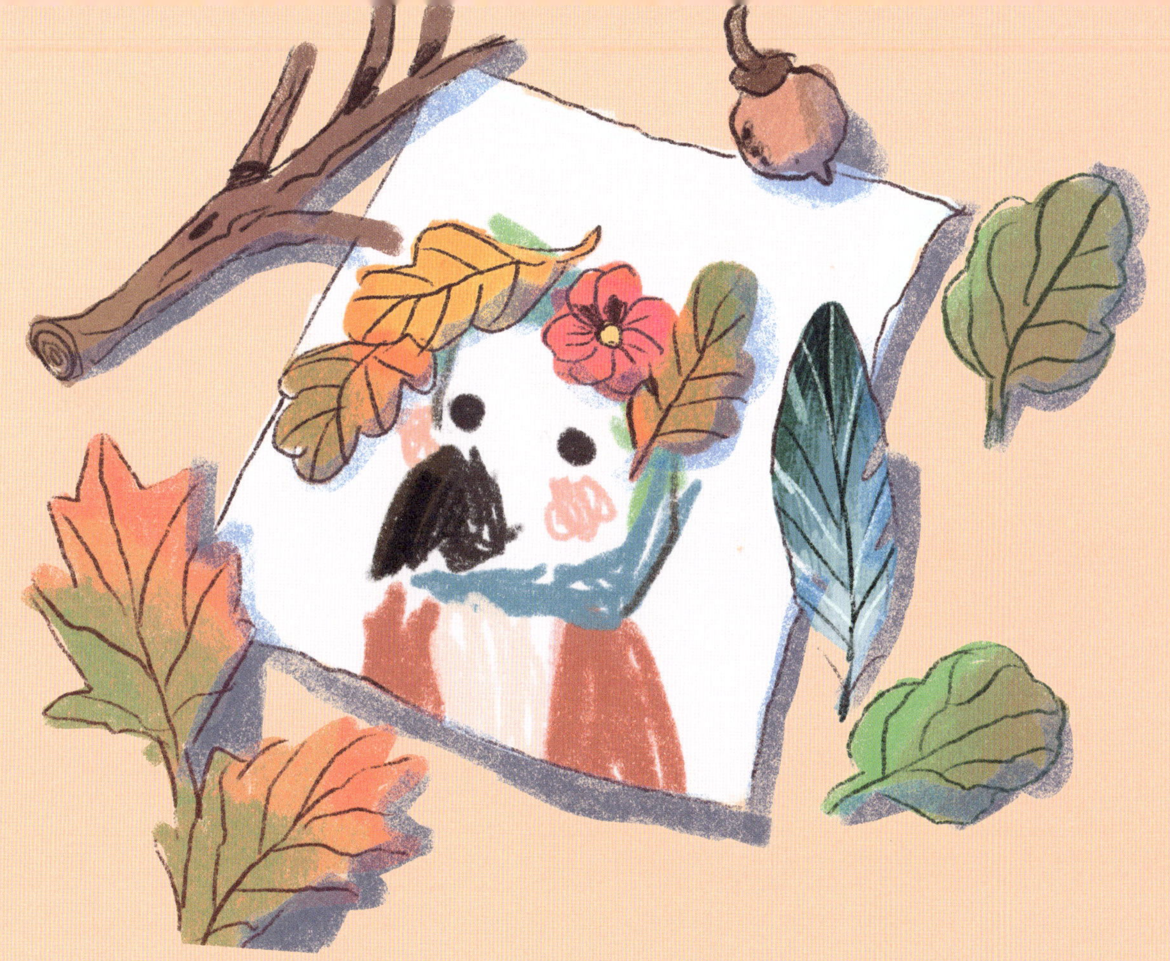

When you get home...

1. Draw an oval on a piece of card.
2. Draw on eyes, a nose, and a big smile.
3. Use the things you have found in nature to make hair. Glue them on carefully.
4. Leave your picture to dry.

You might want to make it look like you or someone you know.

Get giggling

When you laugh your brain releases chemicals called endorphins (en-door-fins) that make you feel happy. Laughing makes your body relax too. This helps you to feel calm.

Did you know? Children laugh about 400 times a day, but adults only laugh about 15 times a day. Adults need to have more fun!

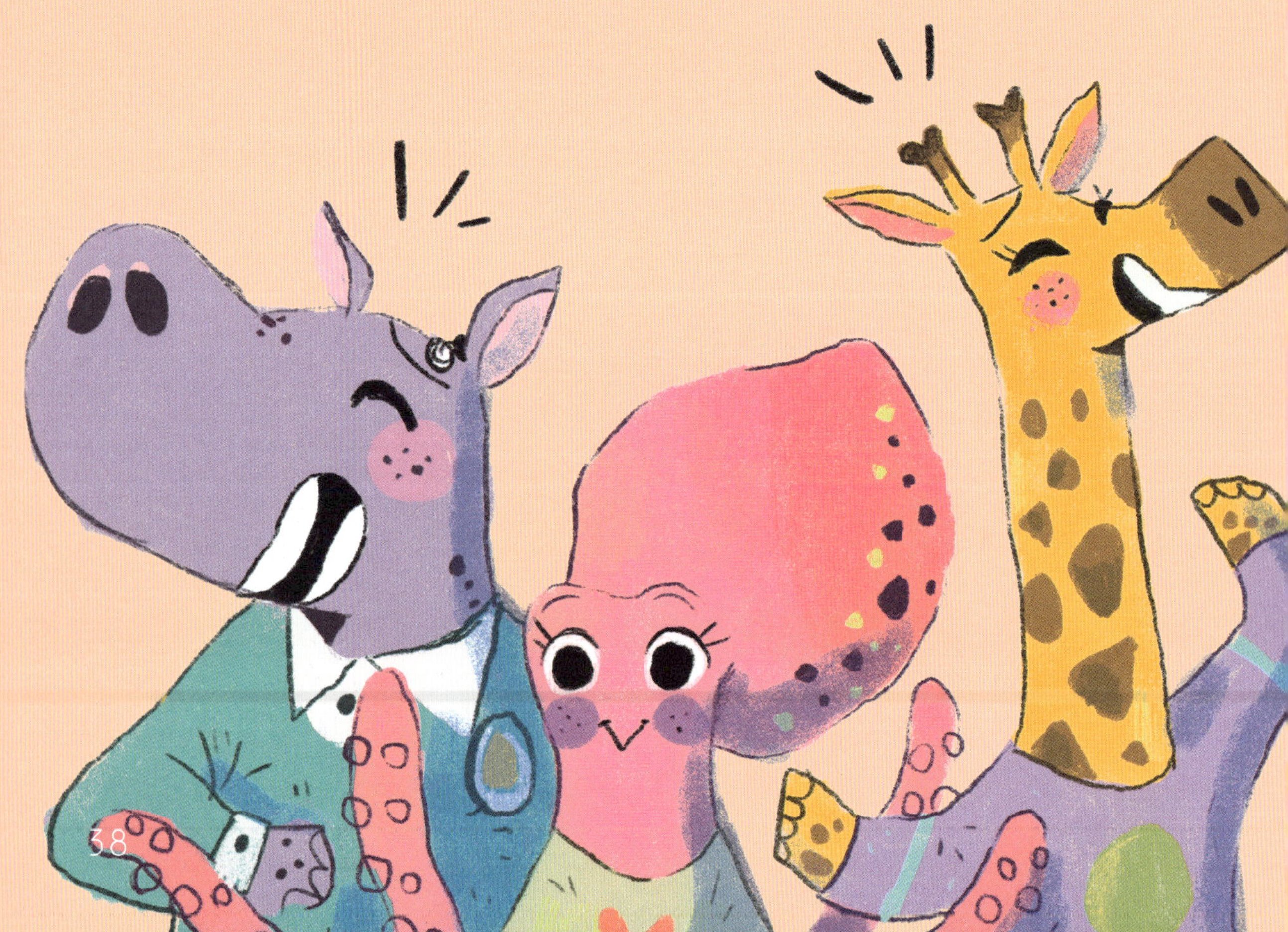

If you want to cheer yourself or someone else up, having a good laugh is a great idea.

What will you try?

Watch a funny movie or cartoon.

Make up fun races for you and your friends. You could walk with teddies on your head or run with a potato on a spoon.

Dress up in your grown-ups' clothes and pretend to be them!

Learn a joke and share it with everyone.

ha ha ha
What's orange and sounds like a parrot? A carrot!

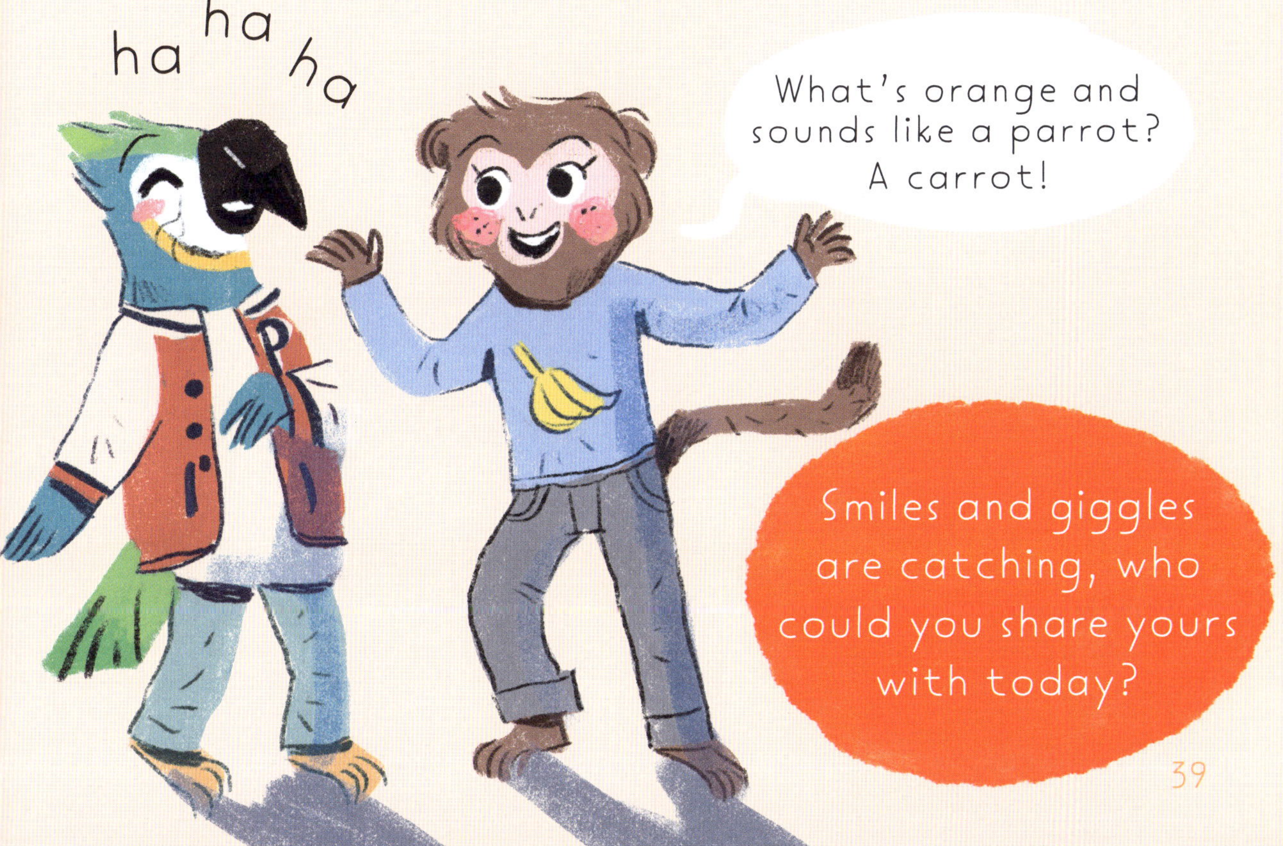

Smiles and giggles are catching, who could you share yours with today?

Make your senses smile

You have 5 senses: smell, taste, touch, sight and sound.

Our senses are amazing and when we make them happy, we feel happier.

Smell

Lots of people like the smell of flowers, cut grass and Sunday dinner.

What smell do you like best?

Taste

Maybe it's bananas, jelly or sprouts that tickle your taste buds?

What taste makes you the happiest?

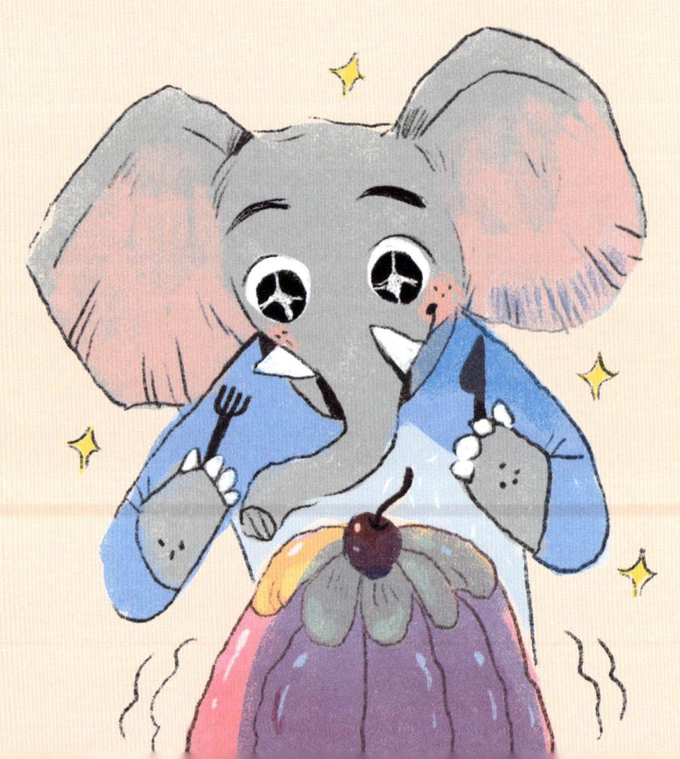

Touch

Maybe you like the feel of a soft blanket or stroking a pet.

What touch makes you feel good?

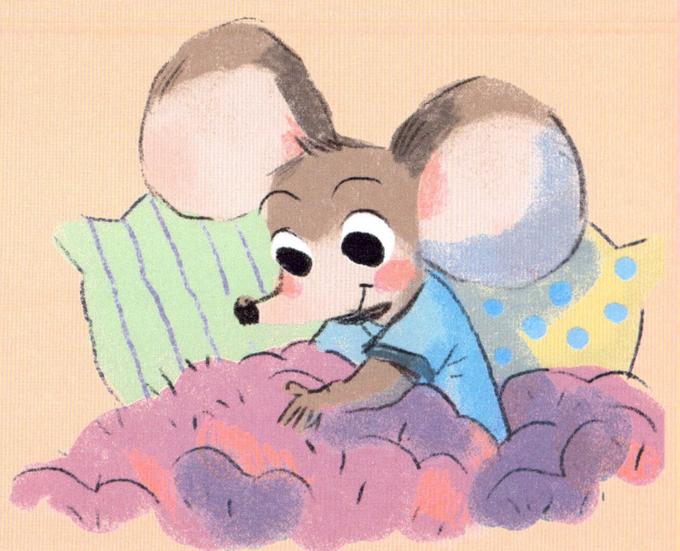

Sight

Some people like to see a rainbow, a friendly smile or the snow.

What sight makes you smile wide?

Sound

Perhaps you like to hear rain falling or an owl hooting.

What's your favourite sound?

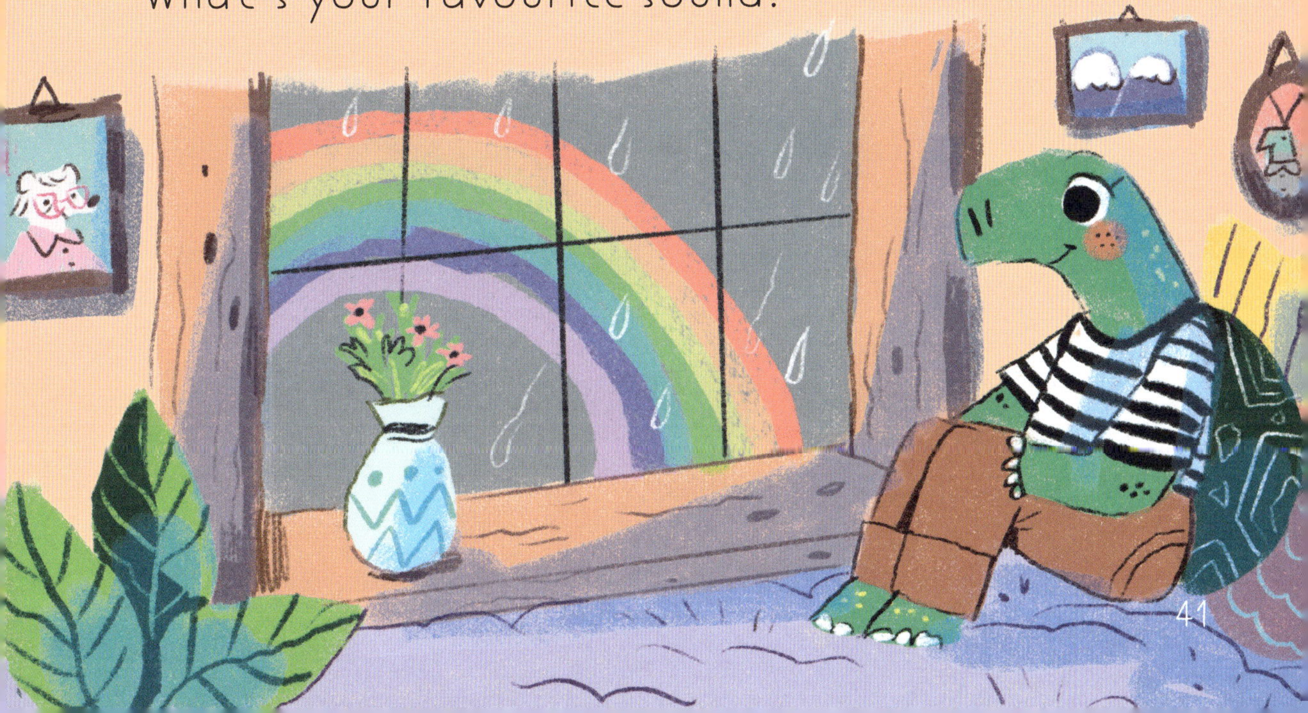

Kinder

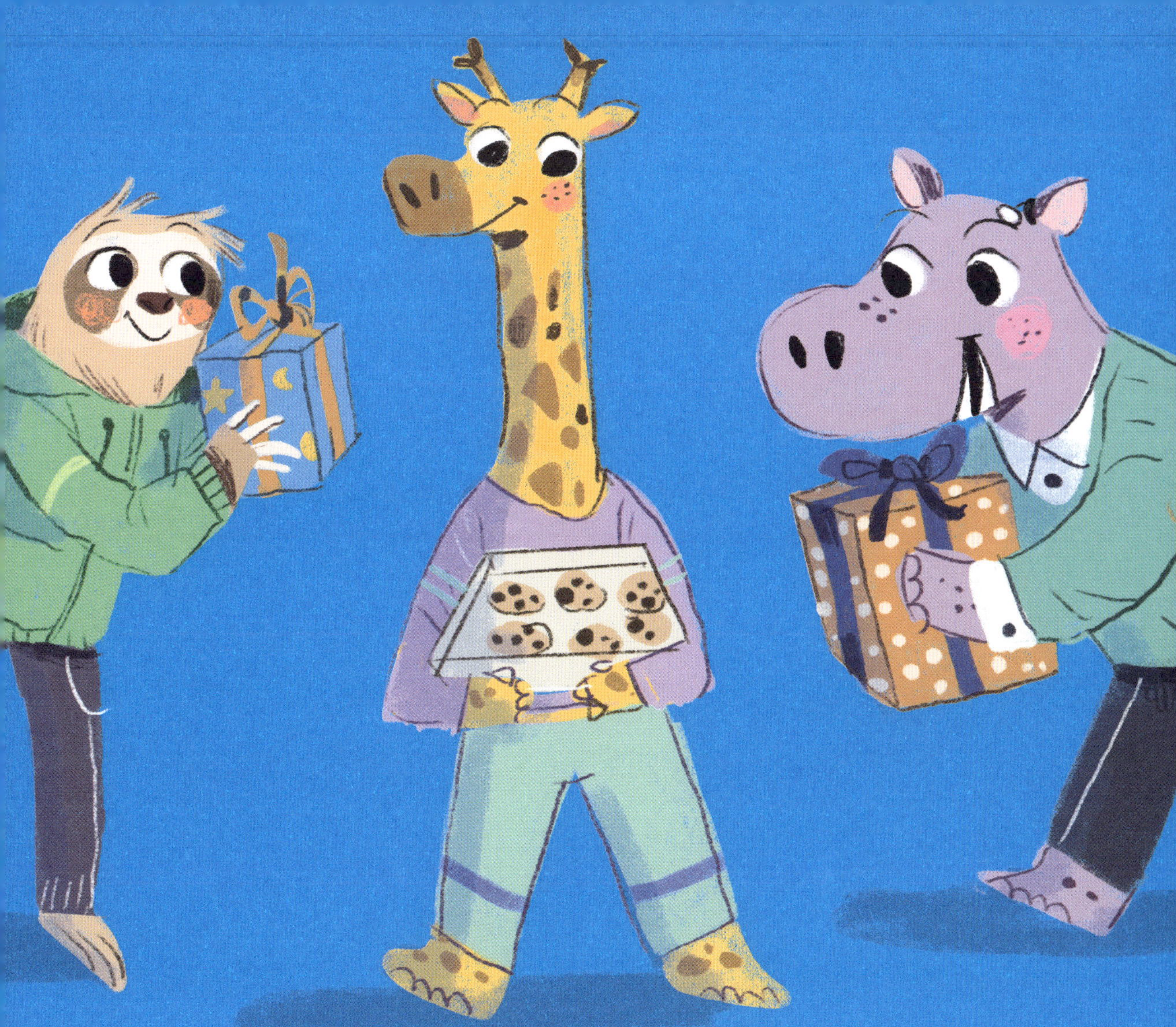

It is so important to be kind.

Being kind to other people makes them feel happy.

Being kind to the planet helps keep it healthy.

Being kind to yourself makes you feel good.

There are many different ways to be kind and they are lots of fun.

Let's take a look.

Share your awesome art

Sharing your art is a fun way to make other people feel happy. When we do nice things for other people it often makes us feel good too.

Window art

1. Make a picture for your window to make people who walk by smile. You could draw your pet, write BOO! or even draw a shining sun.

2. Tape your picture to your window so people on the street can see it.

3. Take a seat and watch how many people enjoy what you have made.

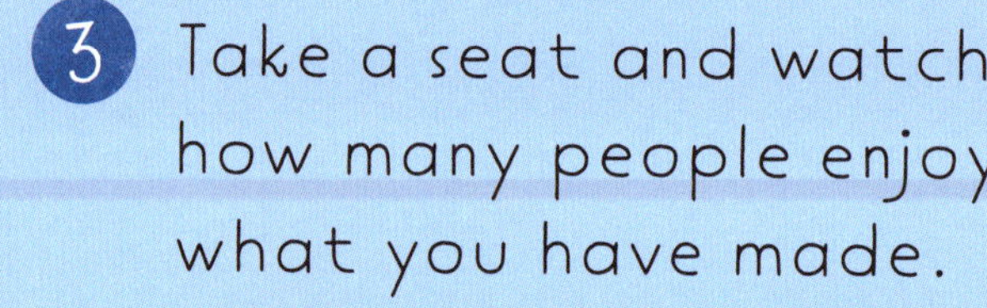

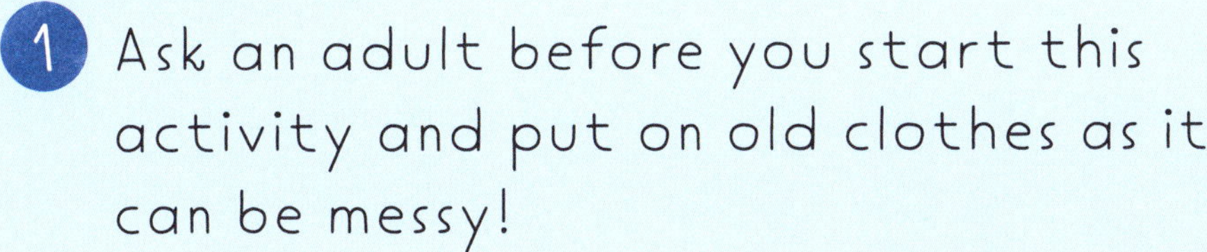

Street art

1. Ask an adult before you start this activity and put on old clothes as it can be messy!

2. Draw a picture on the ground outside your home with pavement chalk. You might want to draw a monster, write Hello or draw a flower.

3. Later take a look outside to see if it makes people smile when passing by.

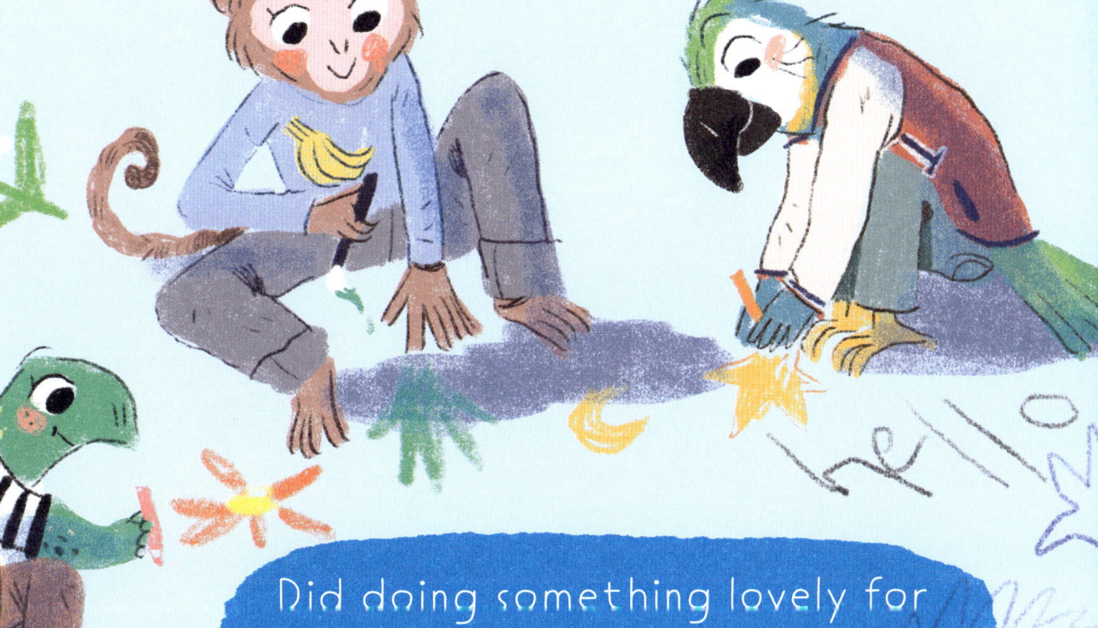

Did doing something lovely for others make you feel happy?

Make a kindness bowl

Making a kindness bowl helps you to practise being kind to yourself.

1. Fill a small bowl with water.
2. Collect some tiny pebbles and put them next to the bowl.
3. Each time you do something kind, caring or helpful drop a pebble into the bowl and say your kind act out loud.

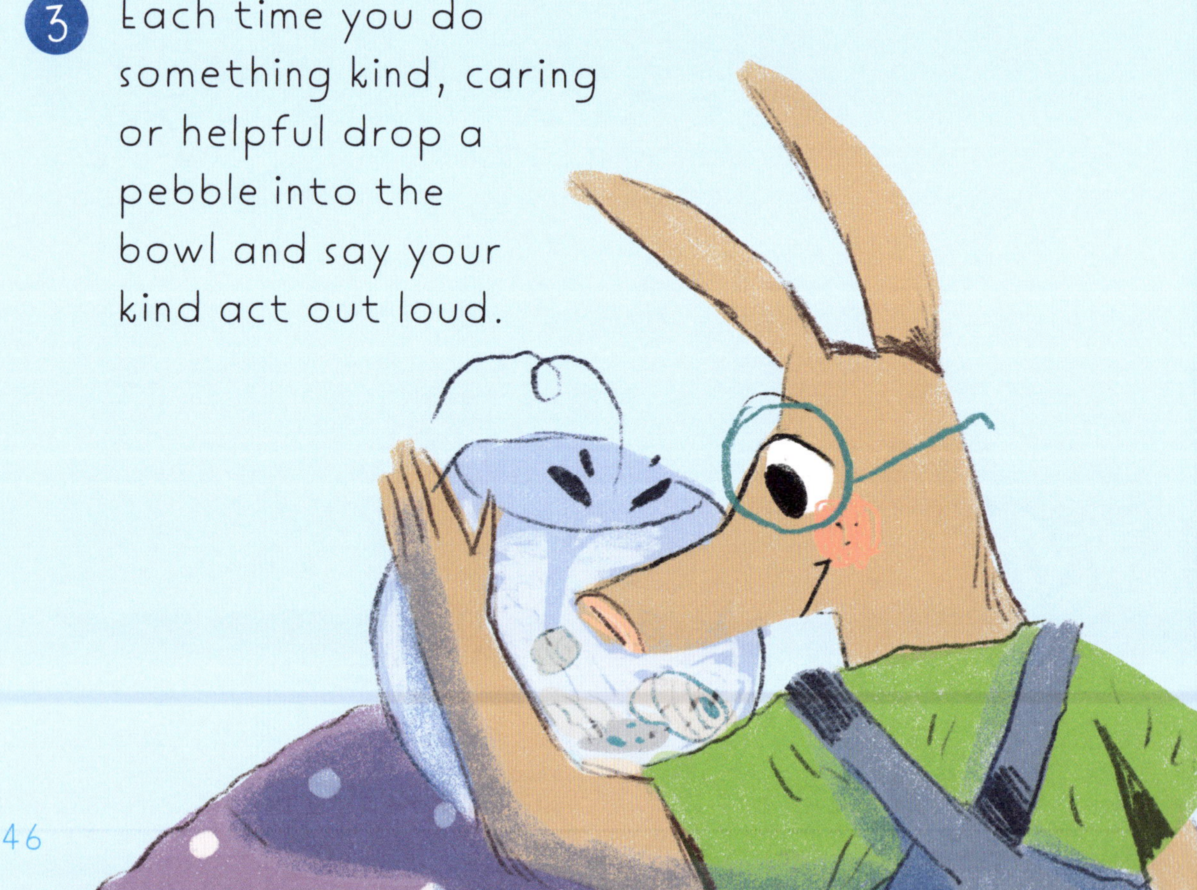

4 At the end of the week pour off the water through a sieve and count up your pebbles to see how much kindness you put out in the world.

You will see lots of ripples when your pebble drops in the water. This shows how kindness spreads too and will remind you of what a big effect it has.

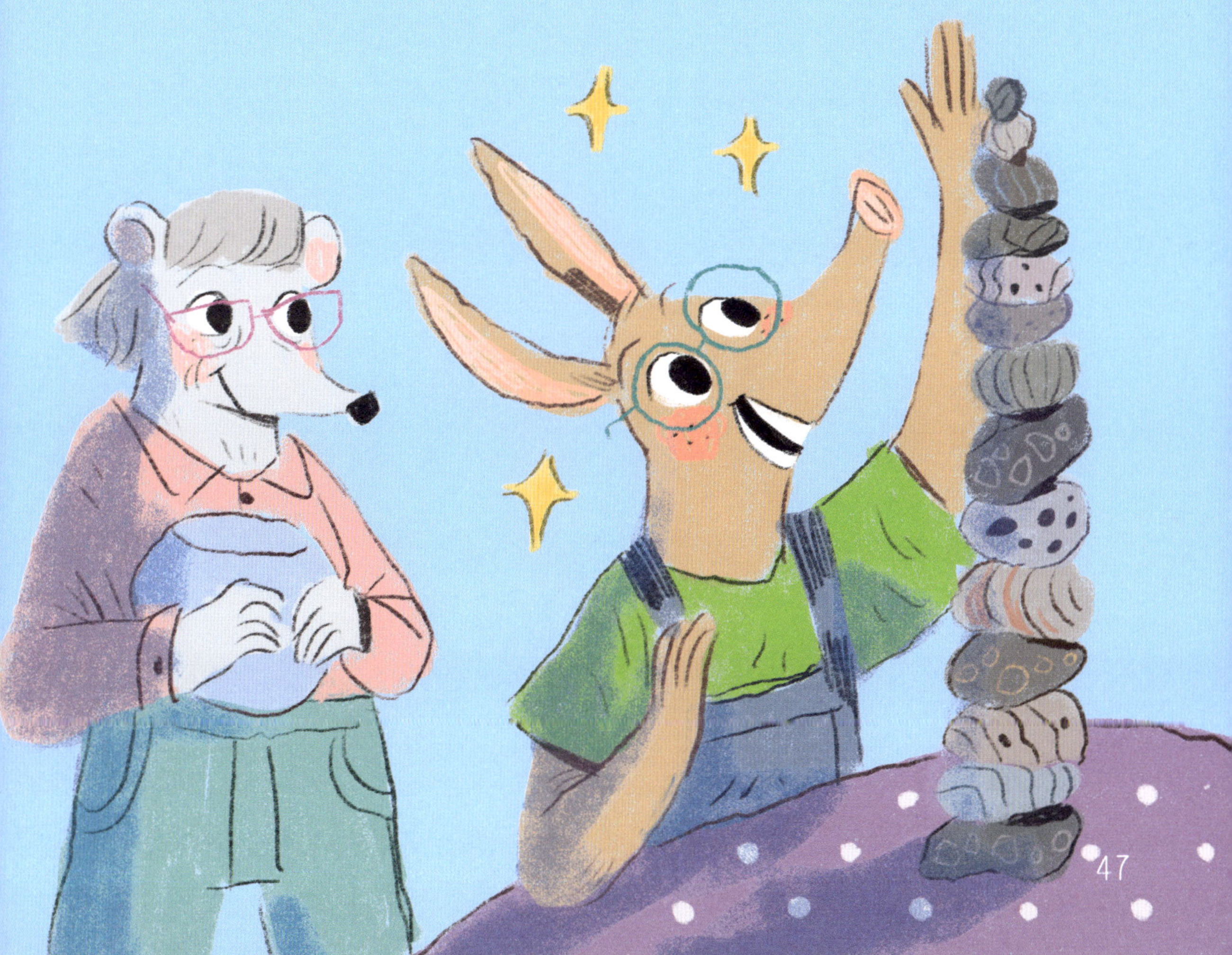

Say something kind

Saying kind words is powerful.

When you say something kind to yourself it makes you feel good. When you say something kind to someone else it makes them feel good too.

Find a mirror to look in and give yourself a big smile. Now say 3 kind things to yourself like...

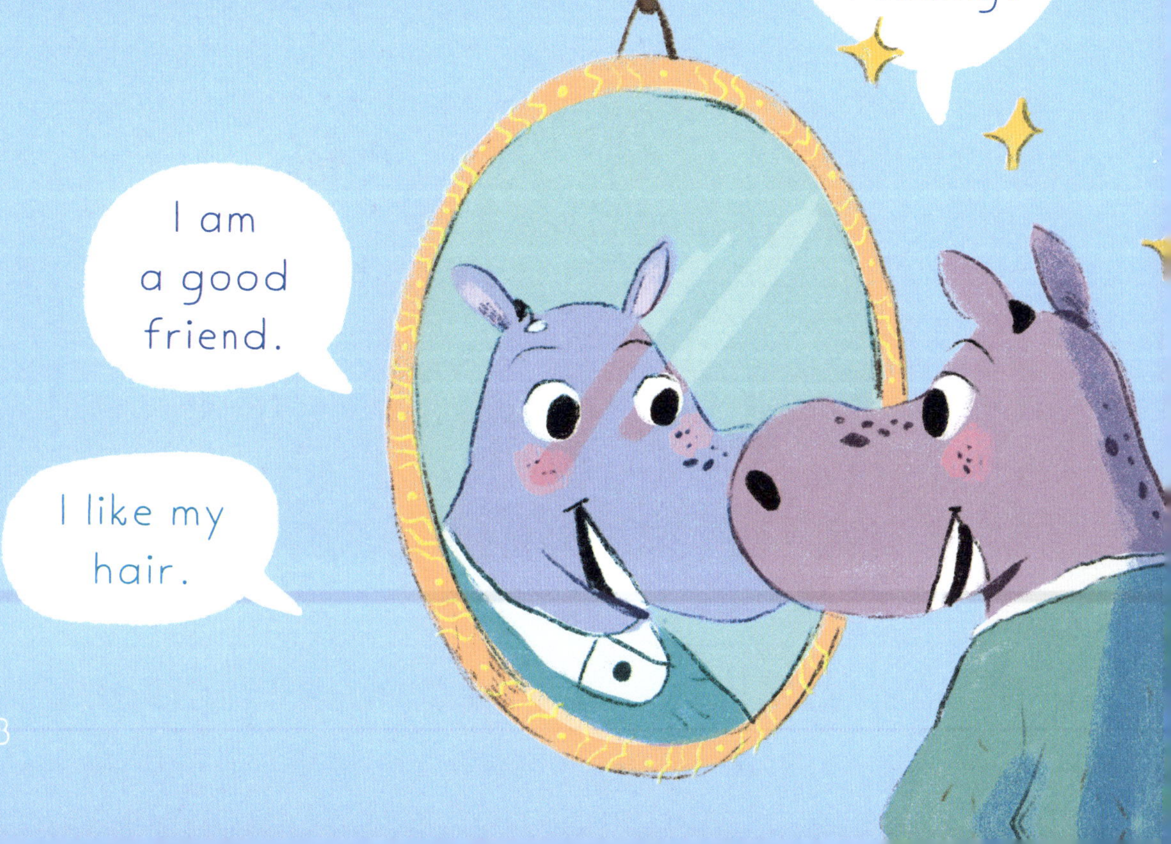

Find 3 people to say something kind to today.
Maybe you could say something like ...

I like your t-shirt.
Would you like to play?
You are so nice.

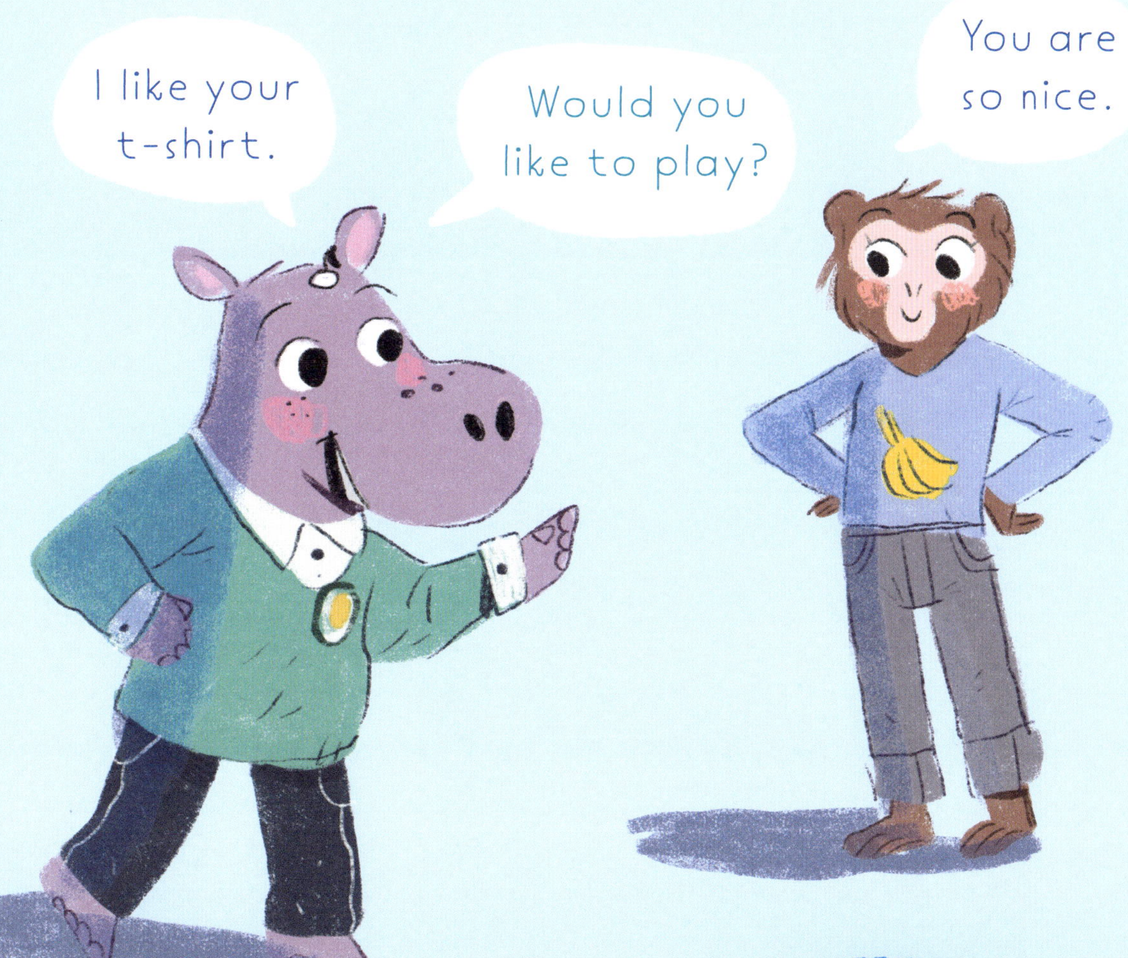

For grown-ups

Let your child overhear you saying kind things to yourself and other people on a regular basis.

If it felt good to say something kind, try doing it more often.

Do animal yoga

A good way to be kind to your body is to take care of it.

Give these fun yoga poses a try and give your body a lovely stretch.

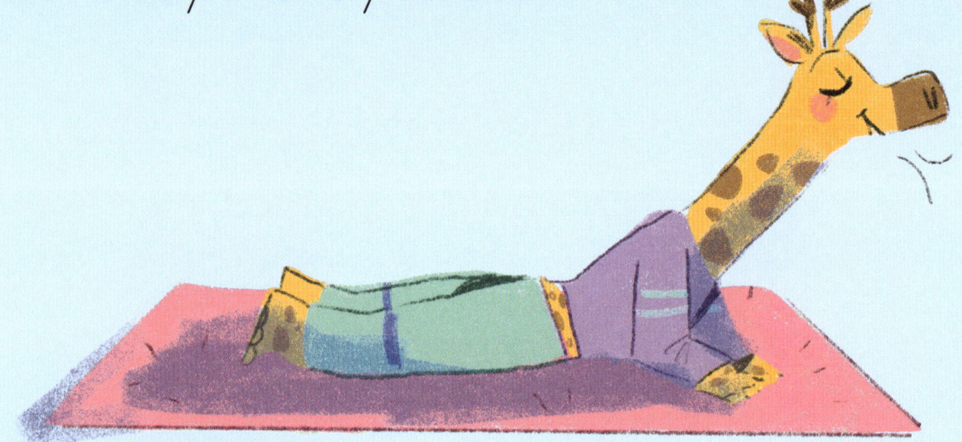

Snake Stretch

1. Lie on your tummy.
2. Put your hands on the floor next to your shoulders, fingers facing forwards.
3. Now push into the floor to lift your head, shoulders, and chest up.
4. Take a big breath in then hiss like a snake.
5. Hold the pose then relax.

Jellyfish Jiggle

1. Lie on your back.
2. Raise your arms and legs slowly into the air.
3. Sway them from side-to-side like a jellyfish in the sea.
4. Do this as you slowly count to 10.
5. Slowly lower them down and sit back up.

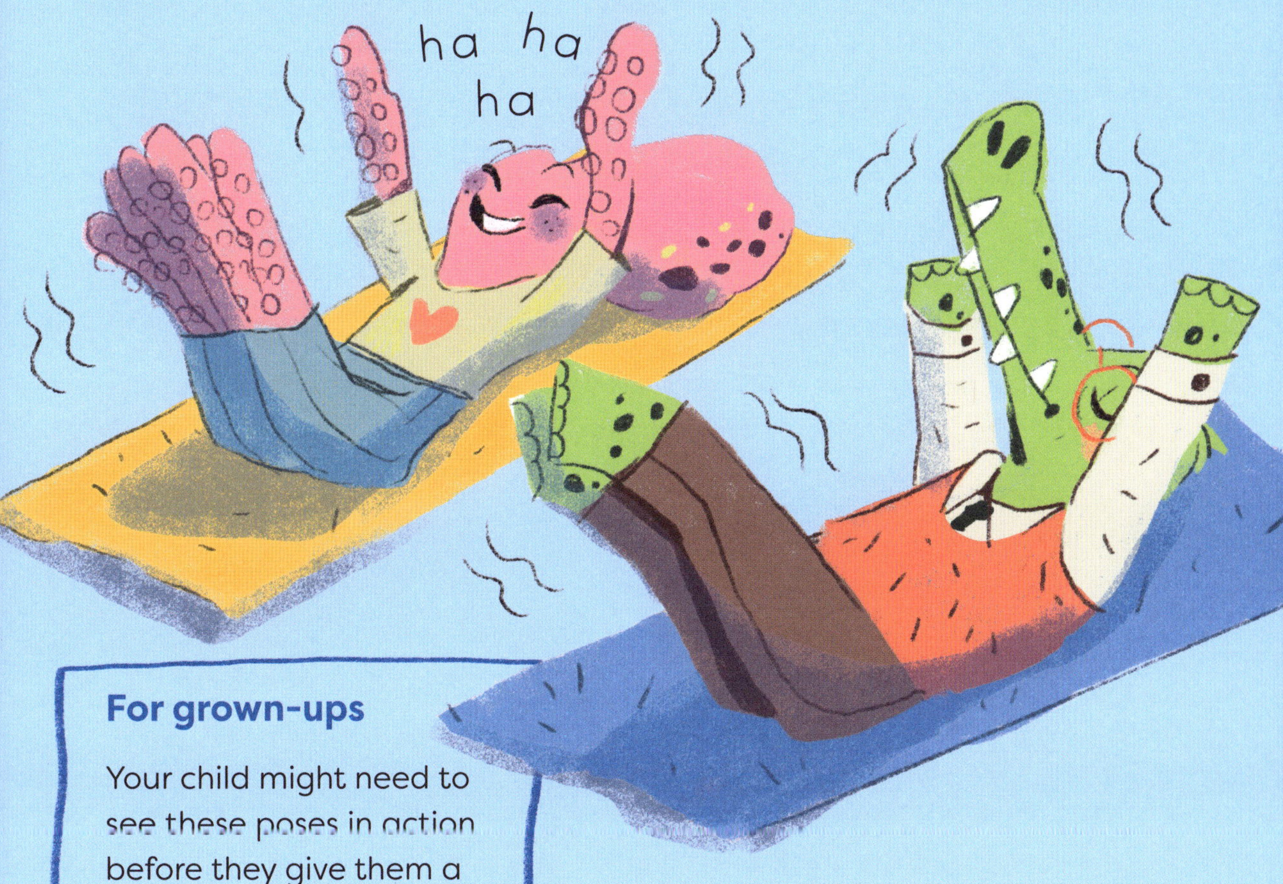

For grown-ups

Your child might need to see these poses in action before they give them a go so do join in!

Make a yummy gift

A homemade gift is one you have made yourself. People like homemade gifts because they show you have put lots of effort into making them.

Making and giving gifts will make you just as happy as the person you give them to.

It's time to get baking!

Easy biscuit recipe

You will need a grown-up helper, an apron and clean hands!

You will also need:

- 100g sugar
- 200g soft butter or vegan spread
- 300g plain flour

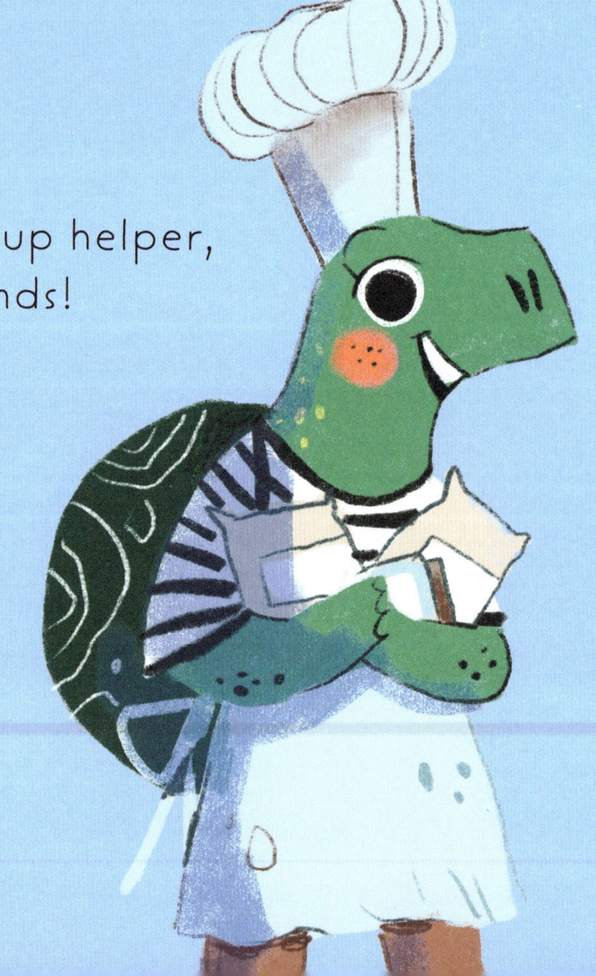

1. Mix the butter and the sugar with a wooden spoon until smooth.
2. Stir in the flour and then use your hands to make a ball of dough.
3. Put a little flour on your worktop and roll out your dough till about ½ cm thick.
4. Cut out shapes with a cookie cutter.
5. Place on greaseproof paper on a baking tray.
6. Put in the fridge for 30 minutes to chill.
7. Pierce each biscuit with a fork and sprinkle them with a little sugar.
8. Bake in a preheated oven at 160°C for 20 minutes.

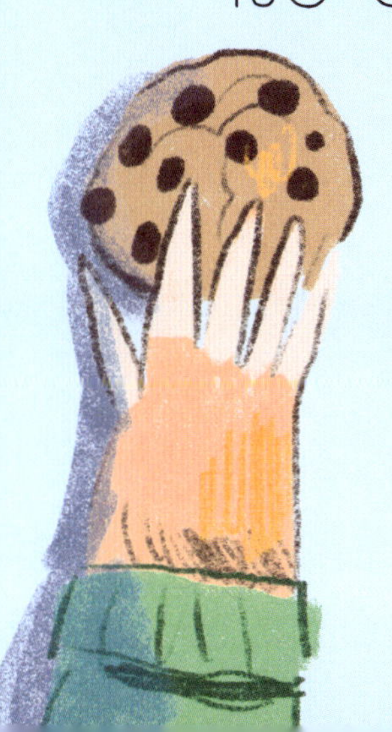

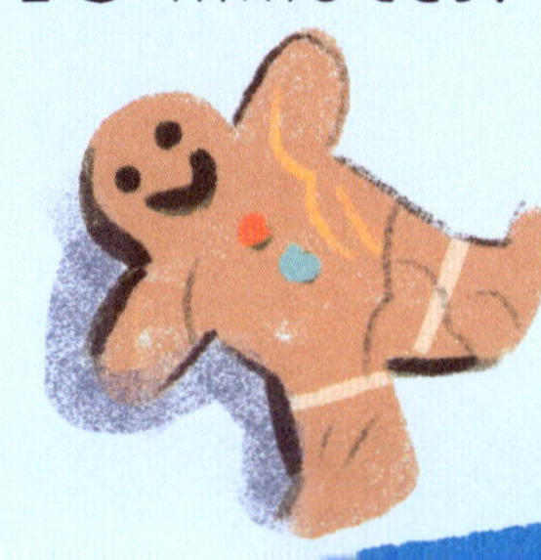

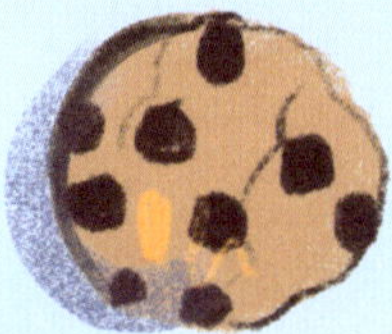

Who could you give your biscuits to?

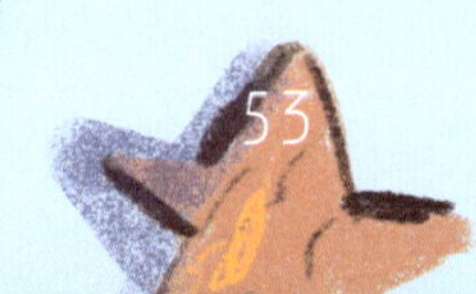

Pass things on

When you don't need or want something anymore it is a great idea to pass it on.

This means someone else gets to use it. Passing things on is much better than something sitting in your house not being used or ending up in the bin.

You will need:

- a cardboard box or a big bag

1. Choose books, toys and clothes that you are happy to give away.
2. Make sure they aren't broken.
3. Put them into your box or bag.

Once your box or bag is full think about who to pass your stuff on to.

Maybe your brother would like your book?
Perhaps your old clothes can go to the charity shop to sell?

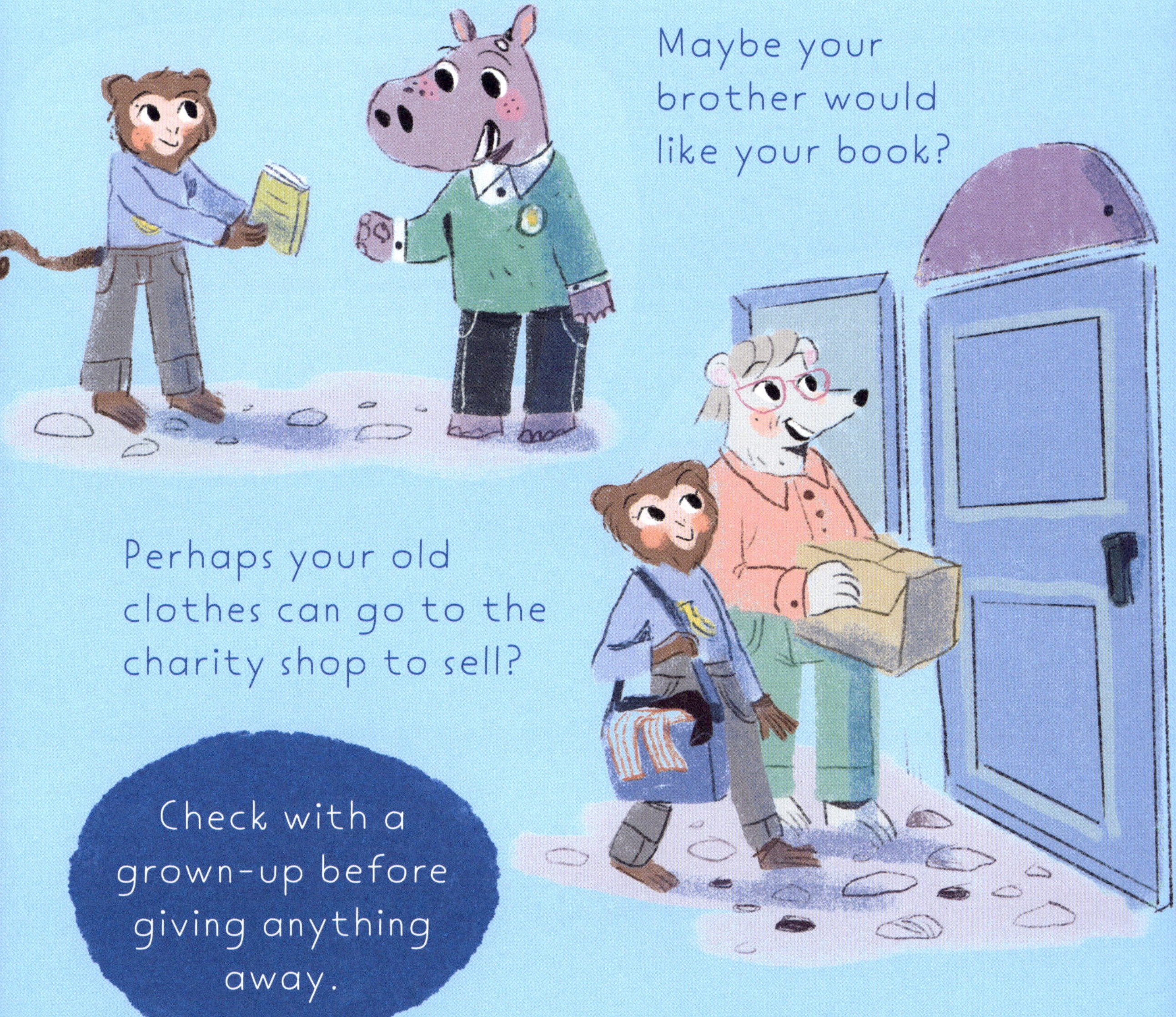

Check with a grown-up before giving anything away.

Passing things on makes other people smile. It helps raise money for charity. And, by not throwing things away, you help the planet too.

Make a friendly fox

The best way to have a good friend is to be a good friend yourself.

Being a good friend means that you are kind, caring, helpful, fun, and thoughtful.

It is good to let your friends know you care about them.

Have a go at making an origami fox to give to one of your favourite friends. Origami (or-i-ga-mee) is making objects by folding paper.

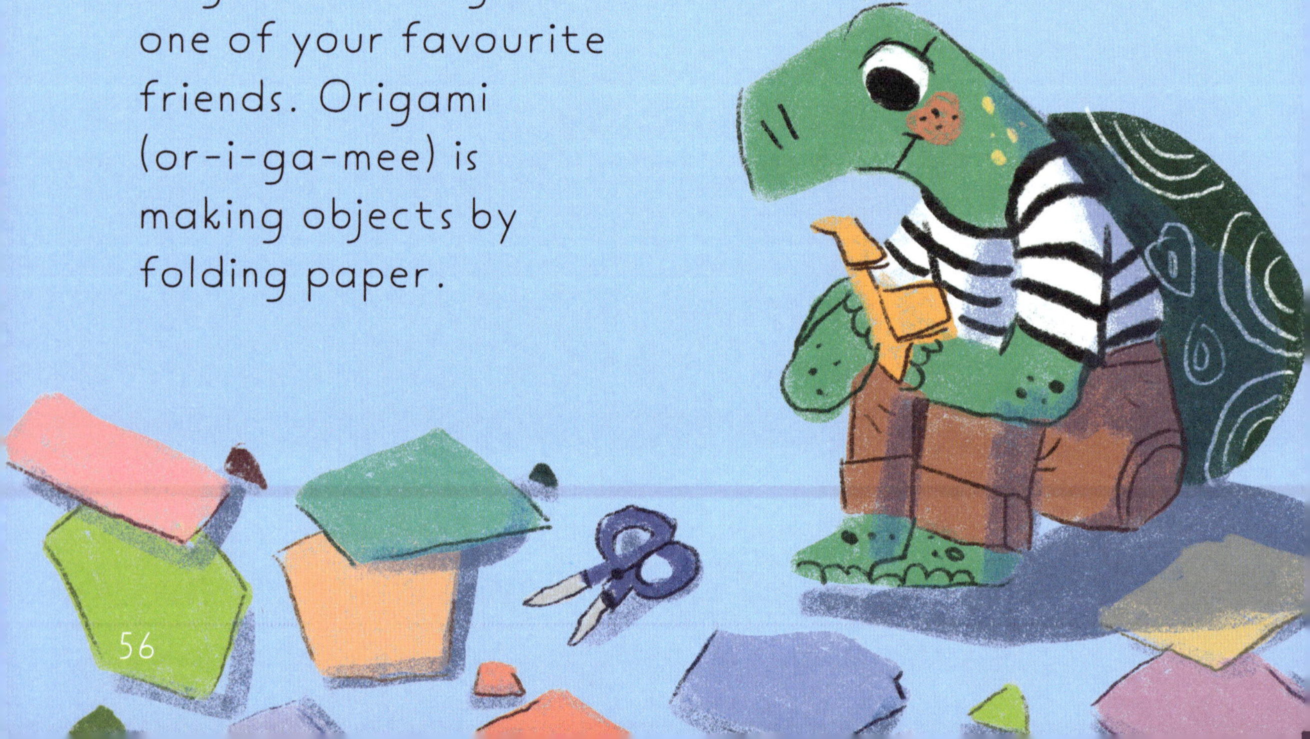

You will need a square piece of brown or orange paper and a black pen.

1 Fold it in half.

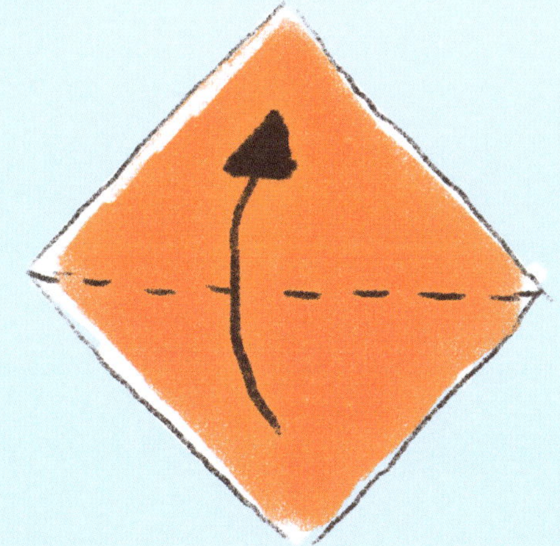

2 Fold down the top of the triangle.

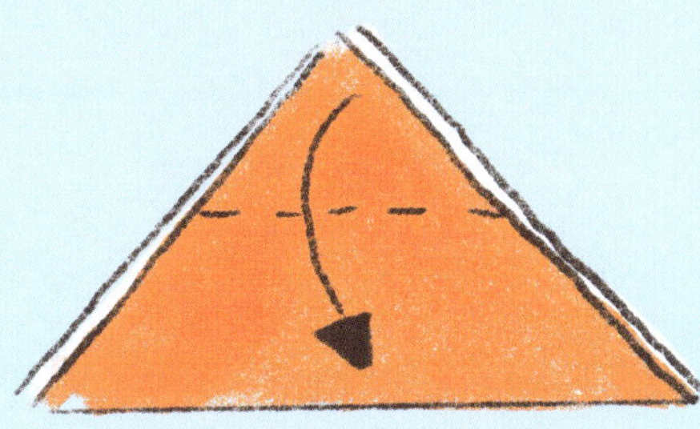

3 Fold up the sides.

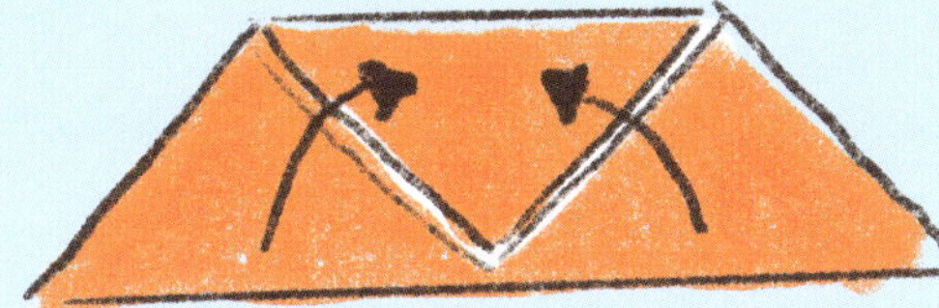

4 Turn your paper over.

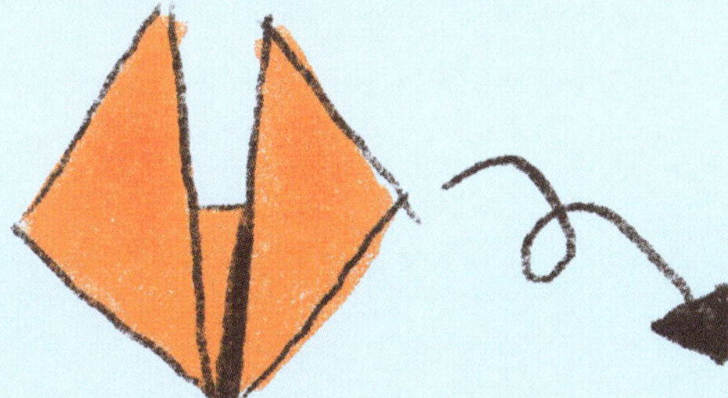

5 Now draw a foxy face.

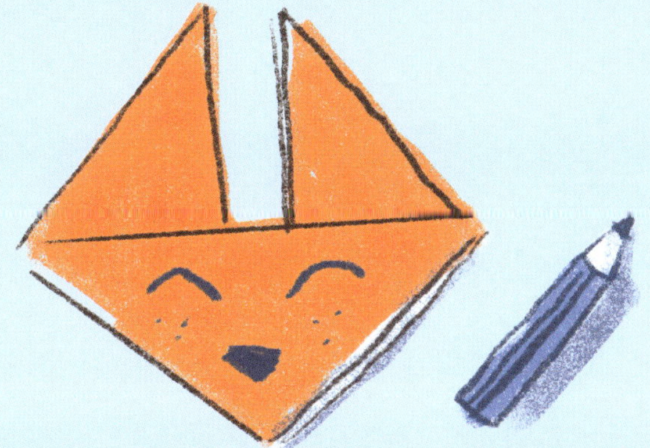

Save the planet

If you take care of the world, it becomes a nicer place to live. There are lots of fun ways to be a planet hero. Here are some ideas you can try...

Go for a walk or bike ride

Do this instead of going out in the car. It will make your legs strong and the planet happy.

Plant something

Look after it whilst it grows. It will need soil, sunshine and water.

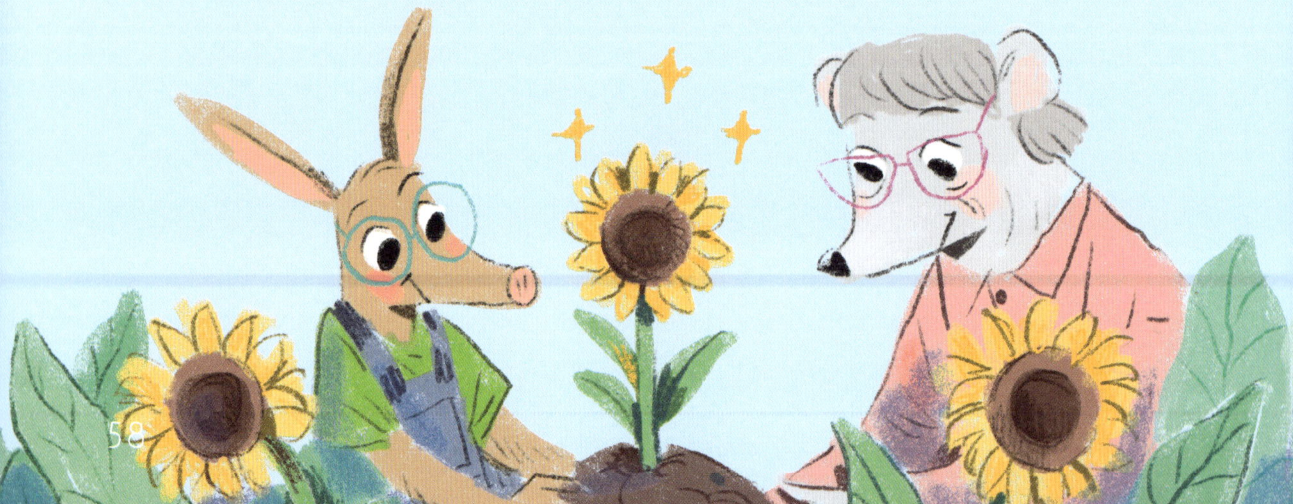

Go litter picking

Don't forget to take a bag and wear gloves. Take a grown-up too!

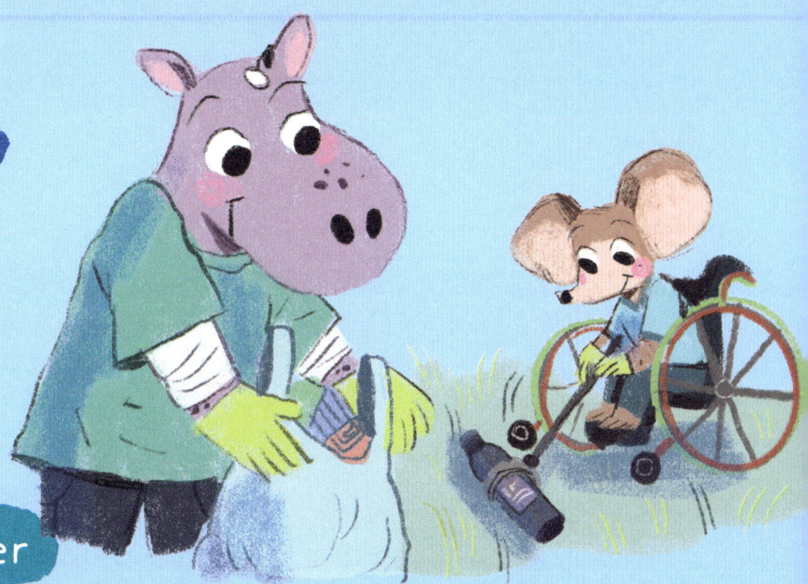

Make a bird feeder

Spread vegetable fat or peanut butter on a pinecone. Roll it in birdseed. Loop string around it and hang it from a tree.

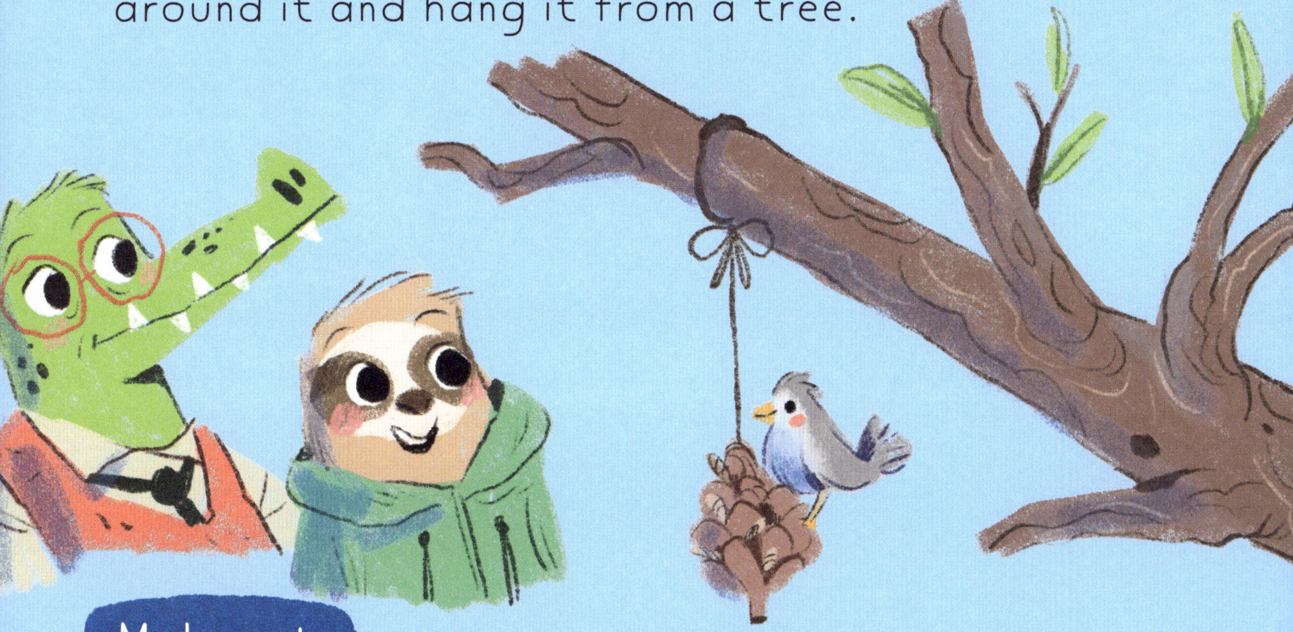

Make art

Instead of throwing away magazines, newspapers and old cards cut them up and use them to make a picture.

Can you think of any more ideas?

Calmer

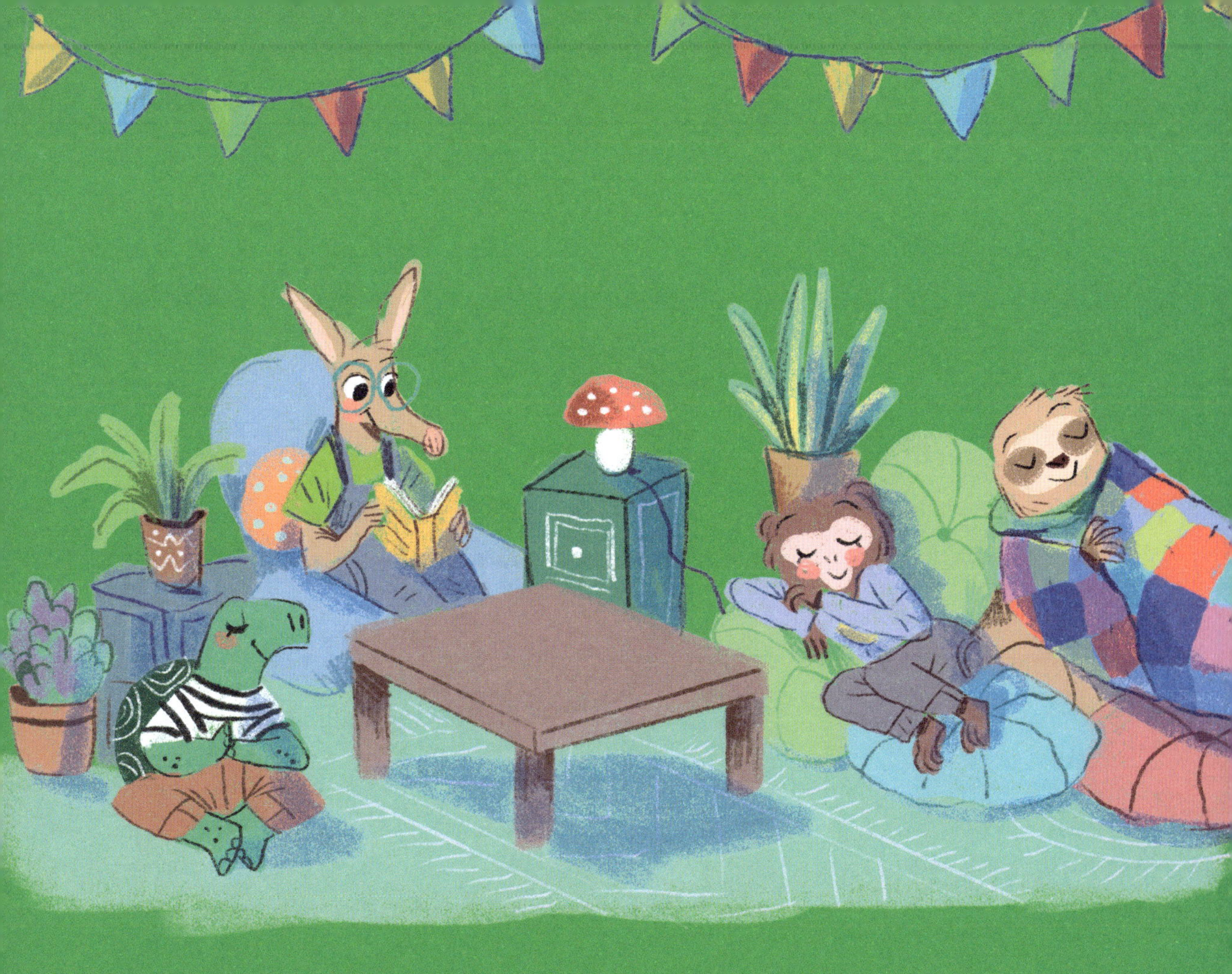

It can be hard to relax when you feel angry or upset. It can be hard to feel calm when you are worried too.

Someone telling you to 'calm down' doesn't always work.

But there are lots of different ways to calm yourself down.

Let's take a look.

Cloud watch (in your head)

Did you know? You can FEEL like you are doing something relaxing just by imagining it.

Isn't that amazing?

For grown-ups

Try reading the instructions to your child in a calm, quiet voice. Doing this activity at bedtime will help build up neural pathways that link bedtime to relaxation. Regular practice will help them to use this strategy themselves in the future.

Let's give it a try:

1. Lie down with your eyes closed.
2. Take 3 slow, deep breaths.
3. Imagine you are lying on your back in a big green field. You can feel the soft grass under you. The sun is shining, and you feel lovely and warm.

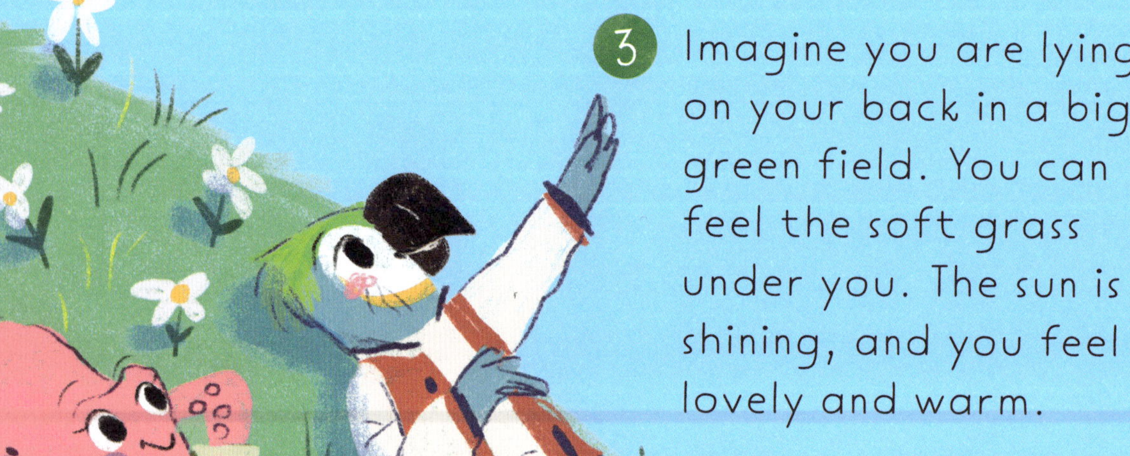

4 The sky is blue above you and there are lots of white fluffy clouds.

5 See the clouds slowly drift along and begin to make shapes.

6 See a heart made out of clouds, then float away.

7 Next, see a tree with big spreading branches.

8 Now see the clouds make a small boat that slowly sails away.

9 You feel very relaxed.

10 When you're ready, give your body a big stretch and gently open your eyes.

Anytime you want to feel calm you can. Simply imagine a calm and happy place and your mood will change.

Try cloud watching outside too. It's great fun.

Feed your worry monster

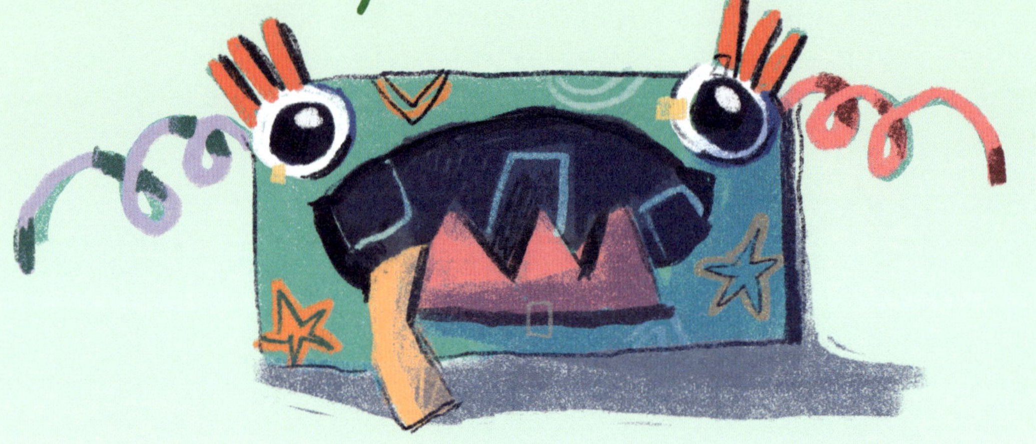

Worry monsters gobble up your worries, so you don't have to keep thinking about them.

You can write or draw what you are worried about, then you can feed the piece of paper to your monster. Feeding your worry monster can help you feel calmer.

If you want, you can look at your worry again later and decide if you want to do something about it.

You will need:

- A tissue box (or any box with a hole in the top)
- Felt tips
- Glue
- Wool or string
- Scissors
- Paint
- Paper

Instructions

1. Paint your box and leave it to dry.
2. The hole in the box is the mouth.
3. You can make teeth for the mouth out of paper.
4. Make eyes using paint or pens.
5. Glue on wool or string for hair.

Don't forget to give your monster a name!

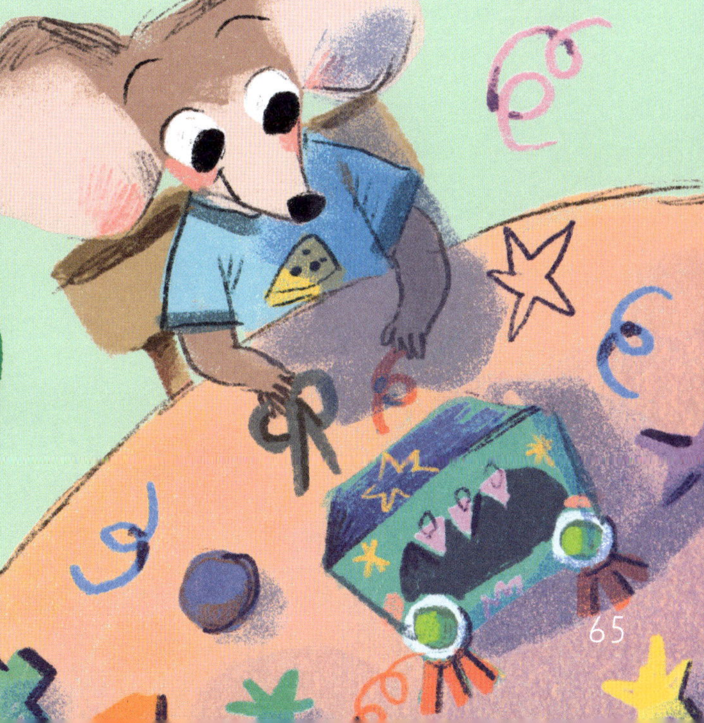

Scrunch it up

When you feel worried, upset, or angry your body might feel tight and scrunched up. This is called tension (ten-shun).

When you squeeze, then relax the muscles in your body, you let the tension go. When your body feels more relaxed your mind will too.

1. Sit quietly on a chair and take off your shoes and socks.
2. Scrunch up your toes. Count 1, 2, 3 then relax and give them a wiggle.

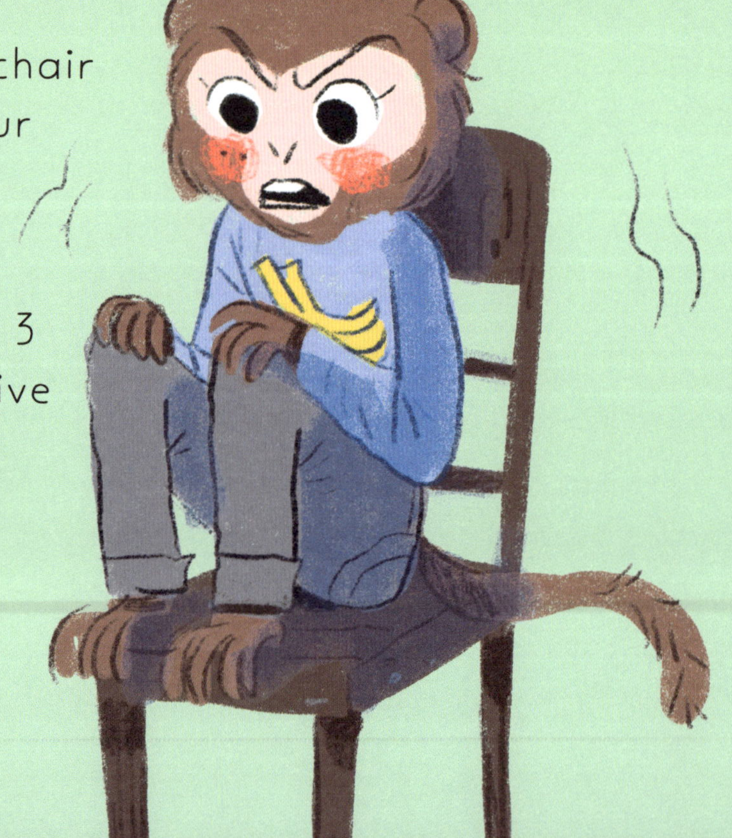

3 Now squash your legs together. Count 1, 2, 3 then let them flop apart.

4 Next pull in your tummy. Count 1, 2, 3 then let it go.

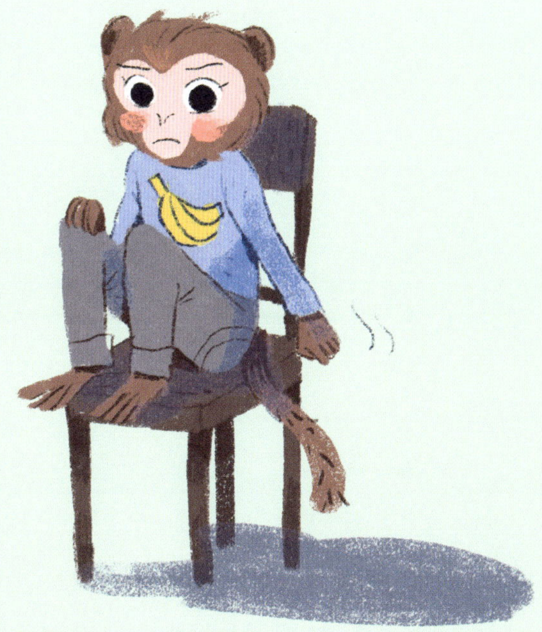

5 Make fists with your hands. Count 1, 2, 3 then spread your fingers wide.

6 Now raise your shoulders. Count 1, 2, 3 and let then them drop.

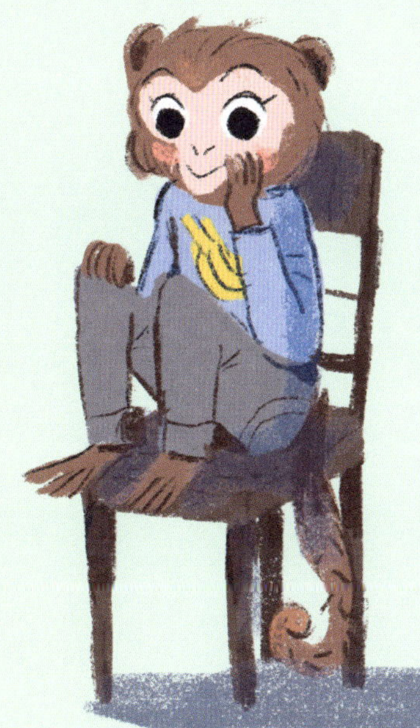

7 Finally scrunch up your nose. Count 1, 2, 3 then smile.

You can do this anytime and anywhere and no one will even notice!

Blow bubbles

When you feel worried or scared your breathing might become fast and shallow and this can make you feel worse.

Taking deep, slow breaths calms your body down. Your body then tells your brain everything is okay and not to worry.

Blowing bubbles is a good way to help you practise taking long, slow breaths.

If you don't have bubbles, you can make your own.

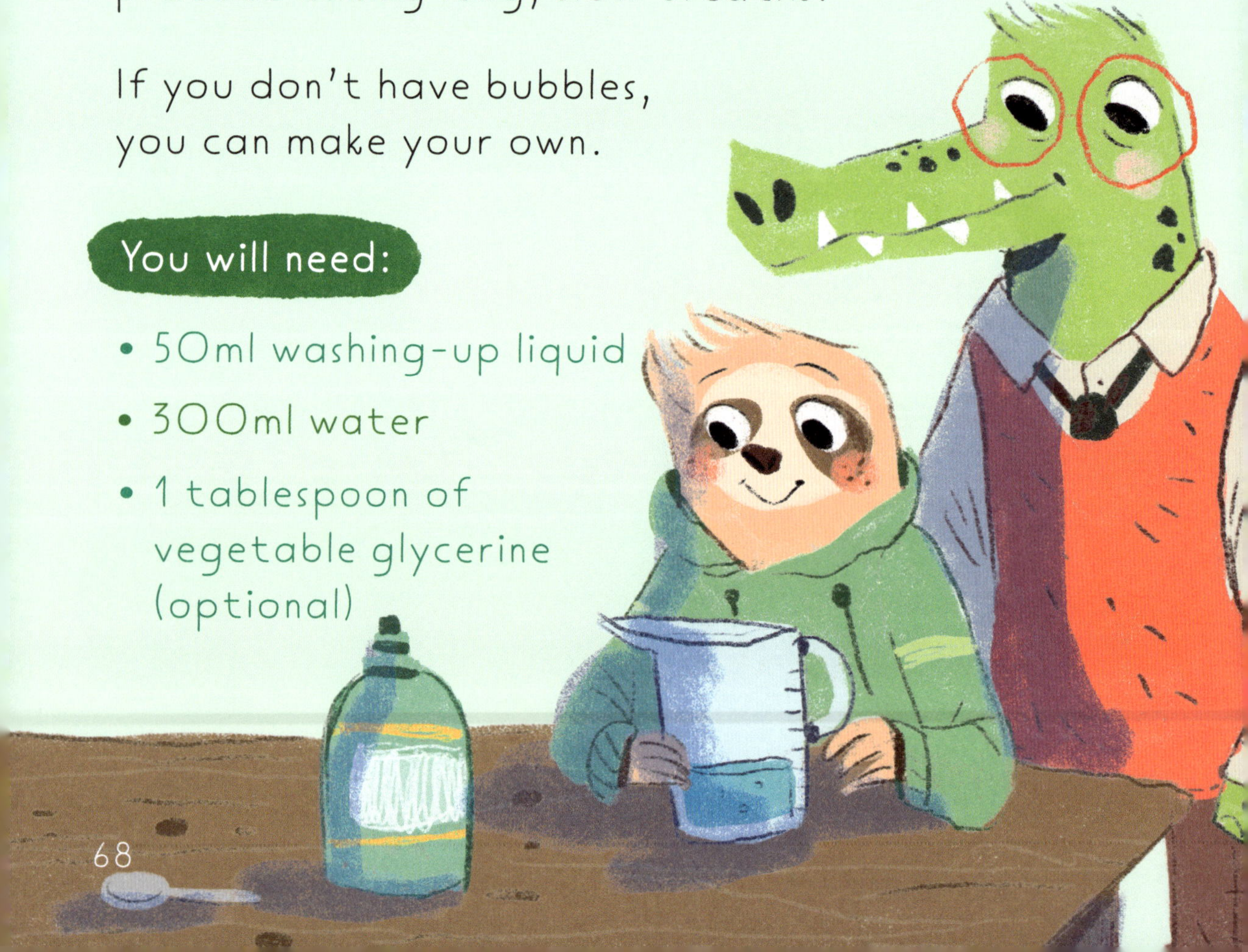

You will need:

- 50ml washing-up liquid
- 300ml water
- 1 tablespoon of vegetable glycerine (optional)

Instructions

1. Pour the water into a measuring jug.
2. Slowly add washing-up liquid and vegetable glycerine and gently stir.
3. Leave overnight.
4. Now your mix is ready to use. If you don't have a bubble-wand, try using a tea-strainer or a slotted spoon.
5. As you blow your bubbles, breathe slowly in through your nose then take a long, slow breath out through your lips.

If you need to calm down and you don't have bubbles then just imagine you do!

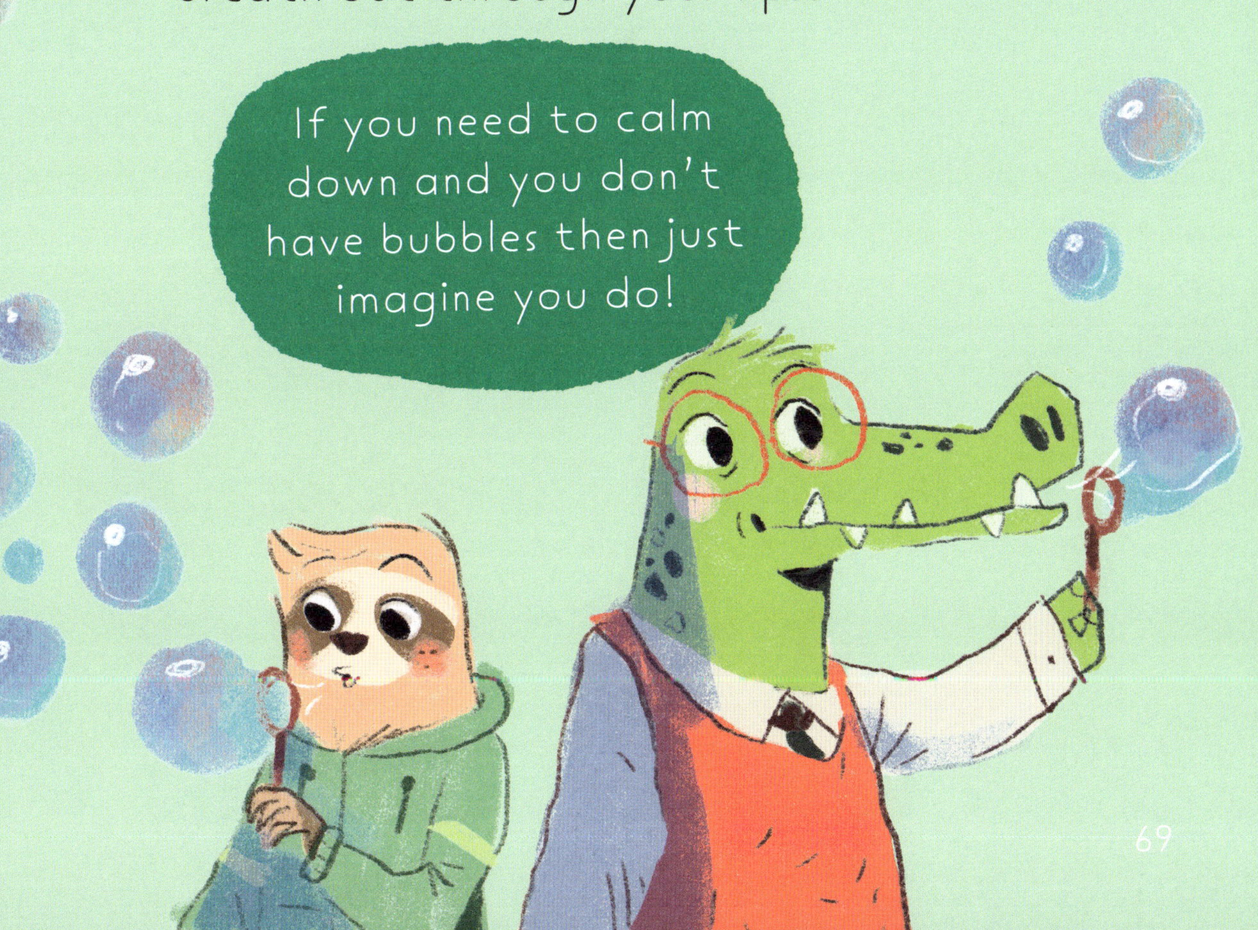

Make a chill-out den

If you feel angry, taking yourself to a quiet place is a good idea. It can help you to feel calm and think more clearly.

Where would you go in your house?

Where would you go at school?

Making a calm-down corner or a chill-out den gives you a great place to go to listen to music, read or just relax.

There are different ways to make a den.

Lay a sheet over the airer

Behind the sofa

Under a table

At the bottom of a bunk bed

Or a sheet over two clothes airers

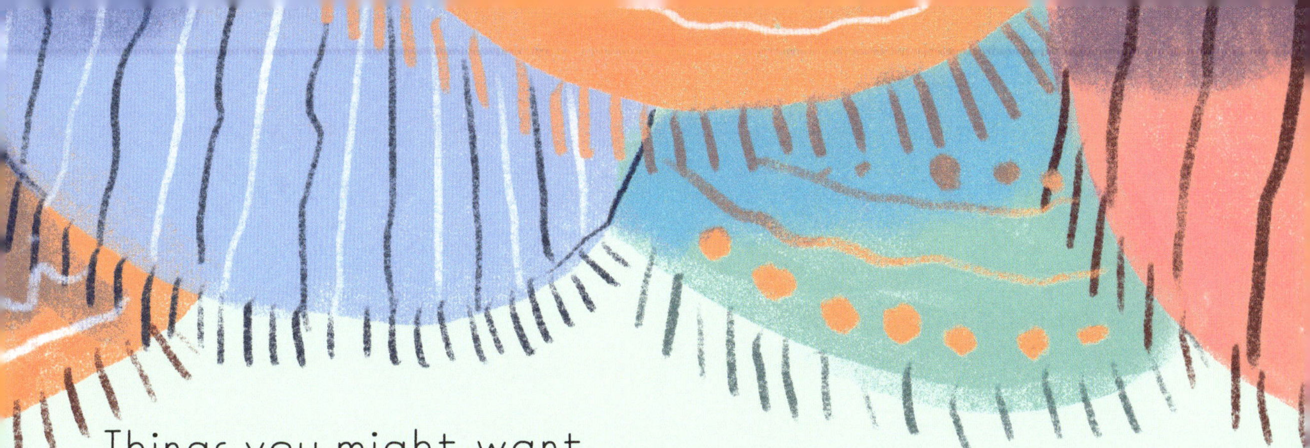

Things you might want to put in your den...

Some toys

Fairy lights

Cushions

A bottle of water

Blankets

Books

Snacks

You might like it so much you never want to leave!

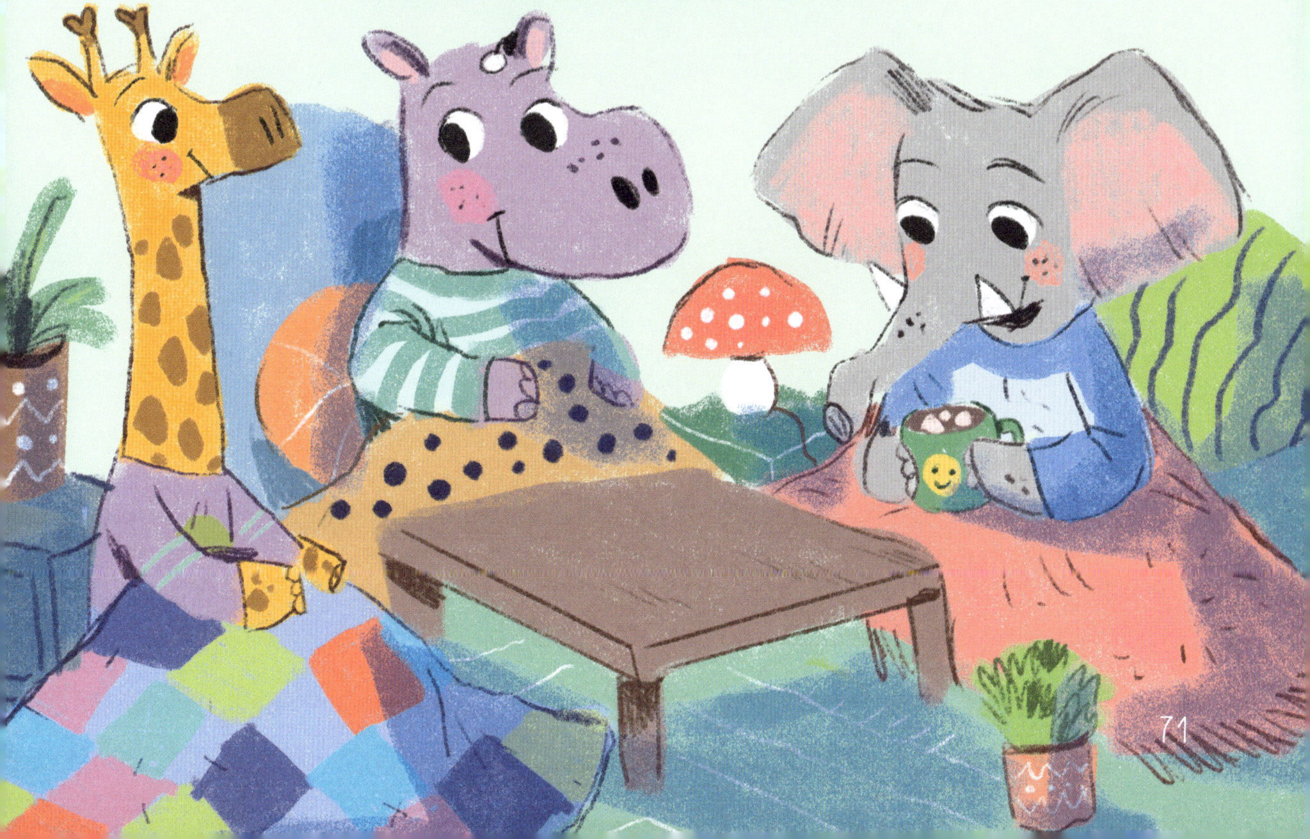

5-4-3-2-1

Looking at and listening to the world around you is called being mindful. It can give you a break from thinking about things that have worried or upset you. This can help calm your mind and body down.

When you are calmer you make better choices about what to do next.

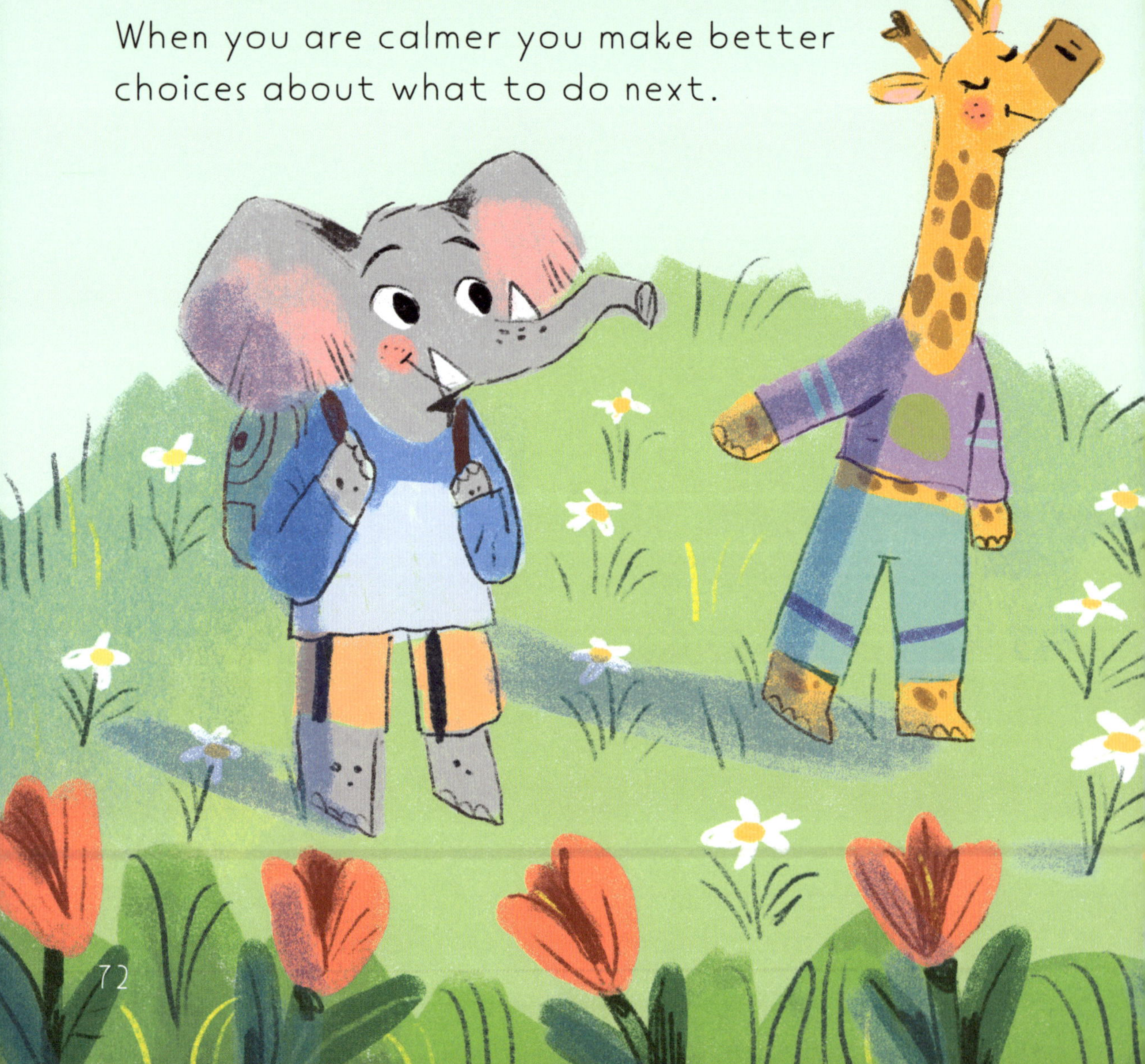

Let's give being mindful a go. Name ...

5 things you can see,

4 things you can touch,

3 things you can hear,

2 things you can smell,

1 thing you can taste.

How do you feel?

For grown-ups

Your child may need you to do this with them a few times until they are able to practise this independently.

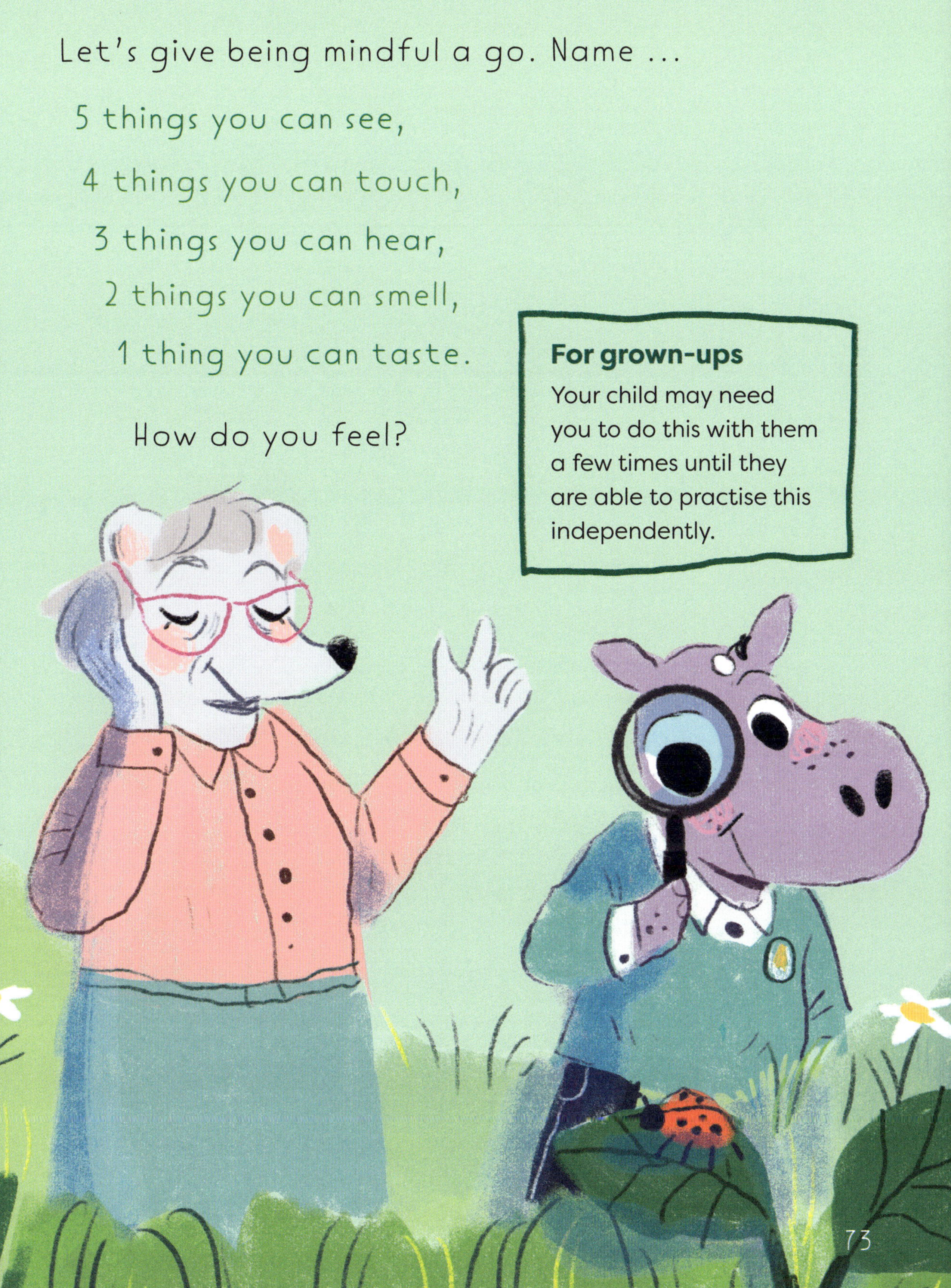

Colour your body

It's okay to feel angry. It's normal. Everyone feels angry sometimes when things feel unfair or unkind.

It's never okay to throw things, hit or shout at people though.

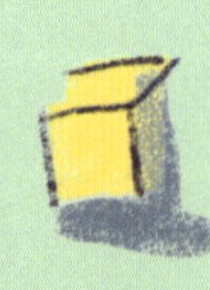

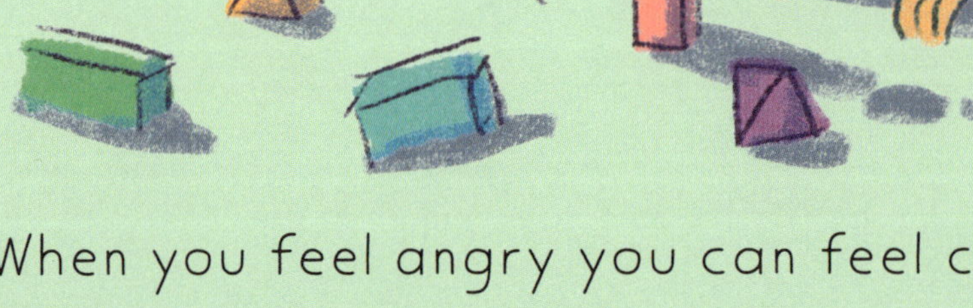

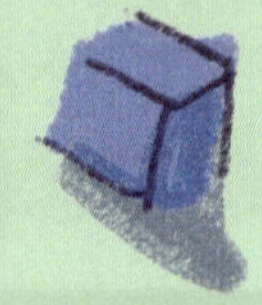

When you feel angry you can feel changes happening in your body. If you notice this happening, you have time to walk away, ask for help or cool down before your anger gets too big.

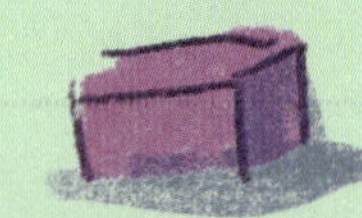

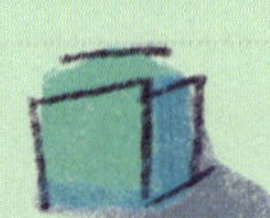

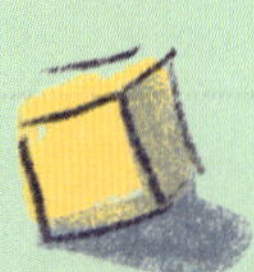

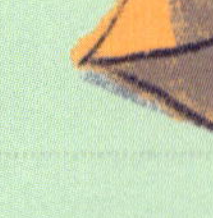

Can you draw a picture of your body and colour the areas red where you might feel anger?

Maybe your ...

Face goes hot and red
Shoulders go up
Heart beats faster
Hands make fists
Tummy feels funny
Legs feel wobbly

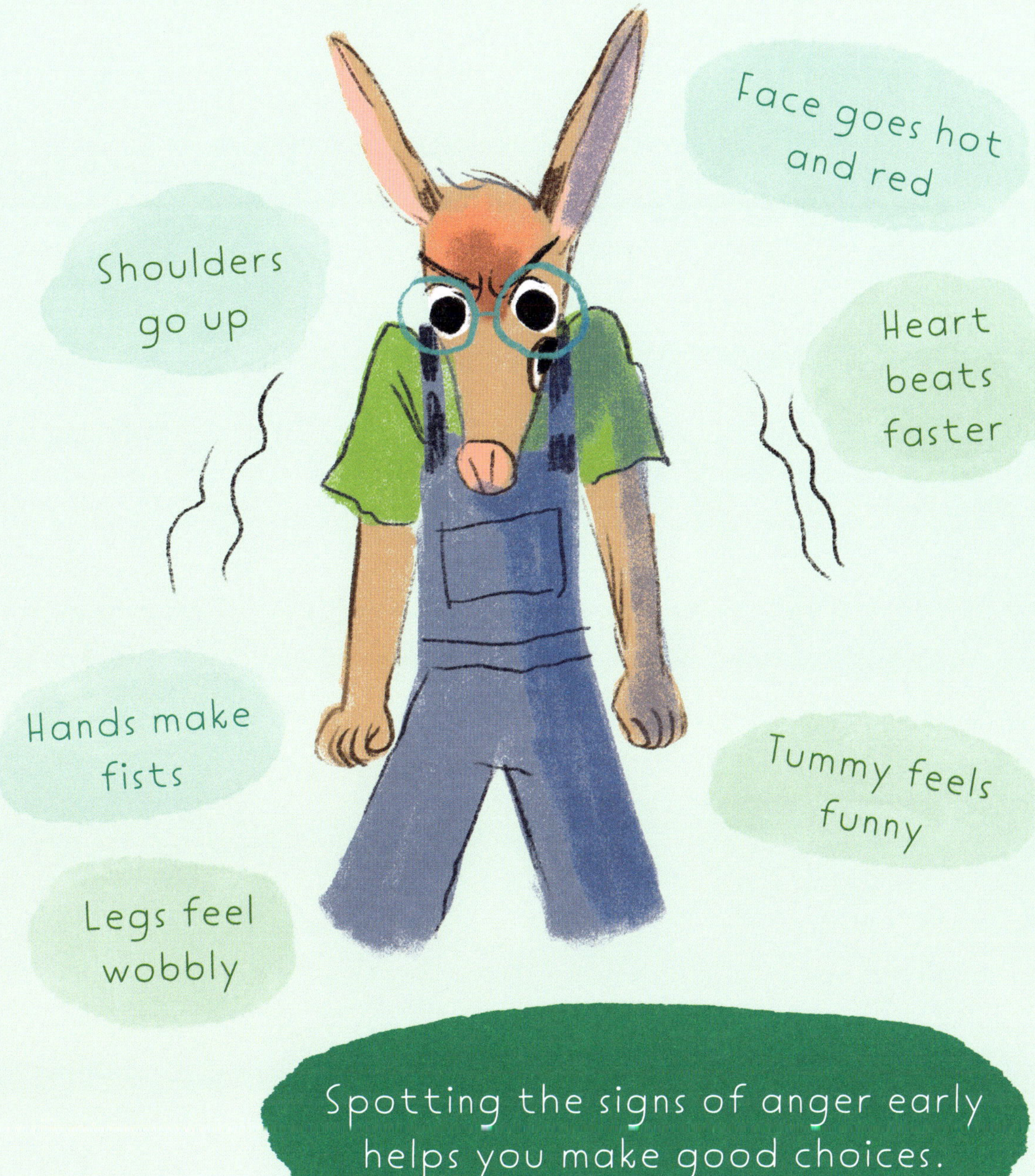

Spotting the signs of anger early helps you make good choices.

Make calm choices

There are lots of different ways to calm yourself down. There is always something you can do that will help.

Have a warm bath

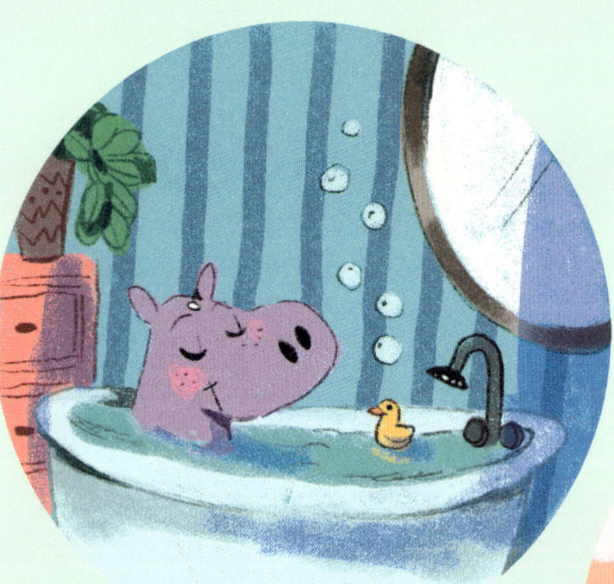

Listen to a story

Do some colouring

Feed the ducks

Snuggle in a blanket

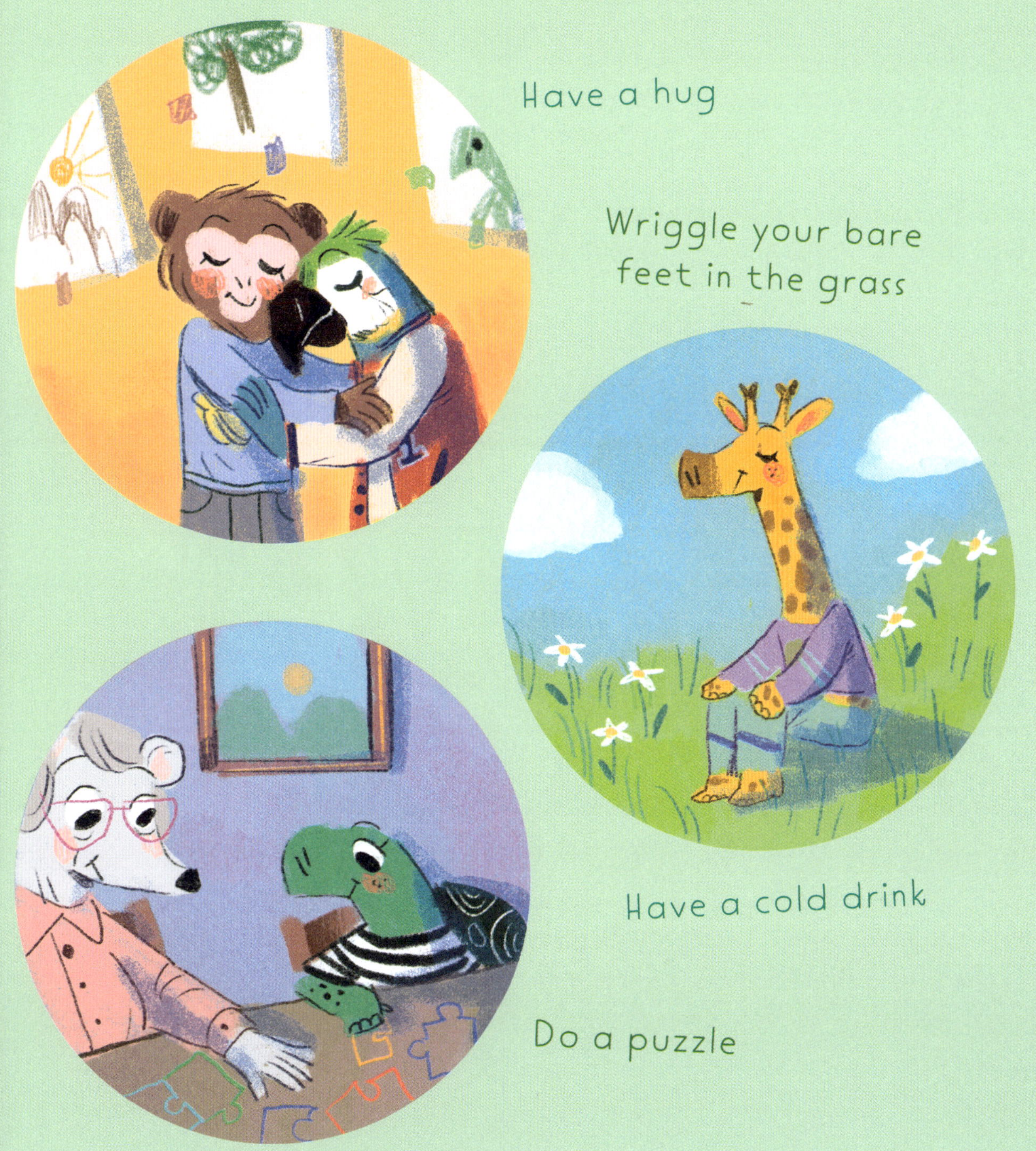

Have a hug

Wriggle your bare feet in the grass

Have a cold drink

Do a puzzle

Pick your favourite way to calm down and use it the next time you feel upset.

Can you think of any more?

Braver

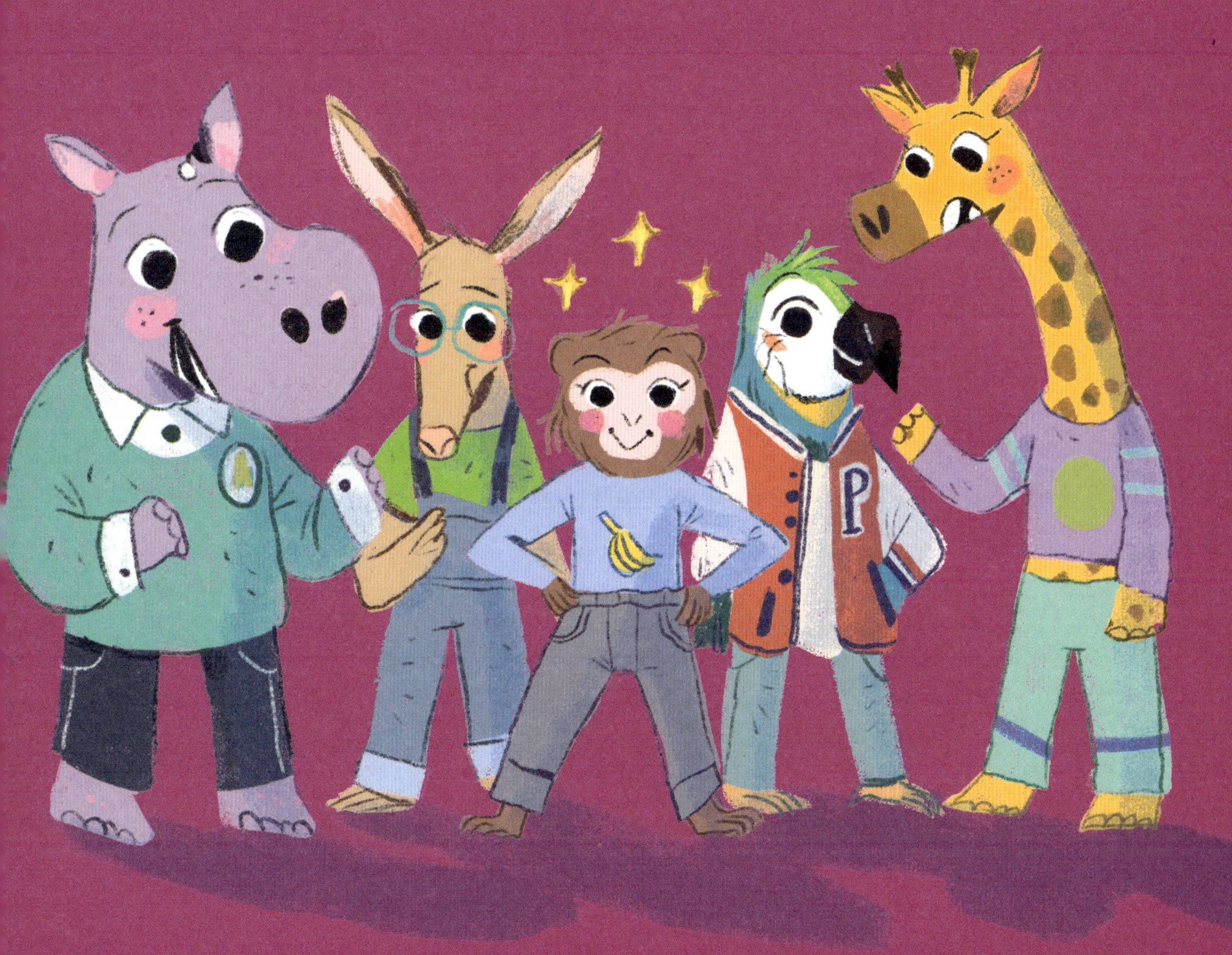

Being brave helps you try new things. It also helps you face things that scare you or have a go at things that seem hard.

If you don't feel very brave right now don't worry, there are lots of ways to become braver.

Let's give them a try!

Tell your bravery story

Think about the jobs firefighters, nurses and the police do. They put out fires, look after sick people and protect people. They have to be brave, every day.

Scientists have found you can catch feelings (like a cold) so, when you think about other people being brave it helps you feel brave too.

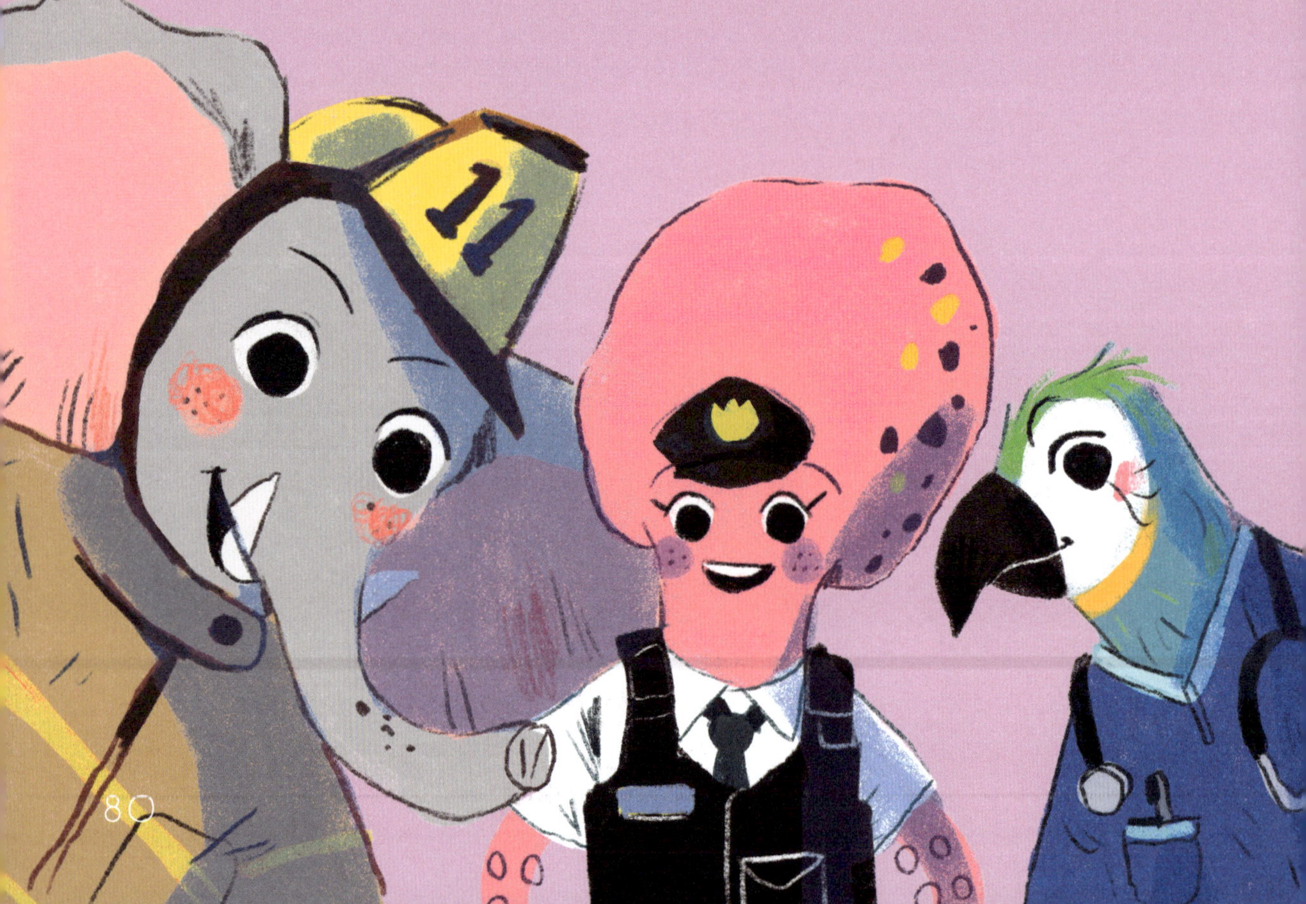

Think about something you did that was brave.

Did you ever fall off your bike while learning to ride?

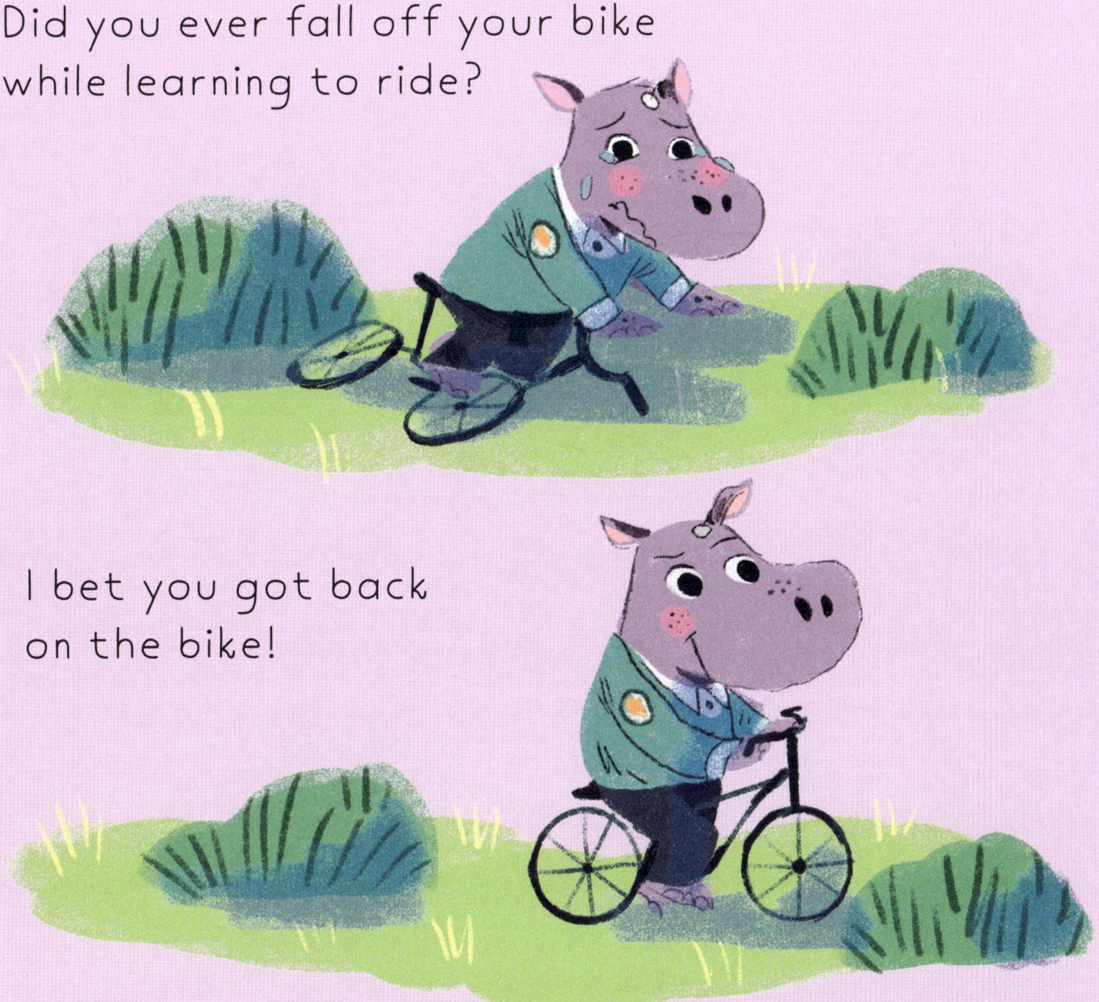

I bet you got back on the bike!

Tell someone your story today or draw a picture of it to share. It will remind you that you can be brave when you need to be and it might help someone else to be brave too.

When you have told someone your bravery story, ask them to tell you theirs. You can inspire each other.

Talk to the mirror

Speaking nicely to yourself can make you feel great.

Scientists have found that if you talk to yourself in a positive way you feel better about yourself and happier.

Choose one of the sentences below and say it three times into the mirror each morning for a week.

I am okay when things change.

I am kind.

I can do hard things.

I am helpful.

I am a good friend.

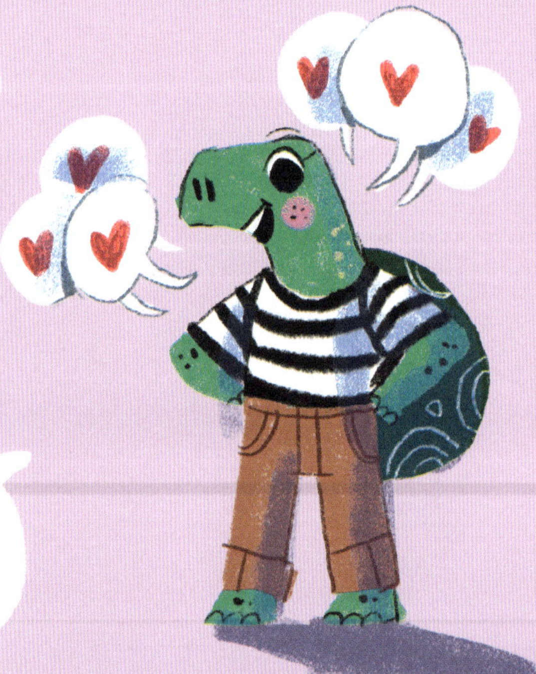

Did you know?

These short sentences are called affirmations (a-fur-may-shuns). They help you to believe in yourself.

This might feel weird at first and it's okay if it makes you laugh.

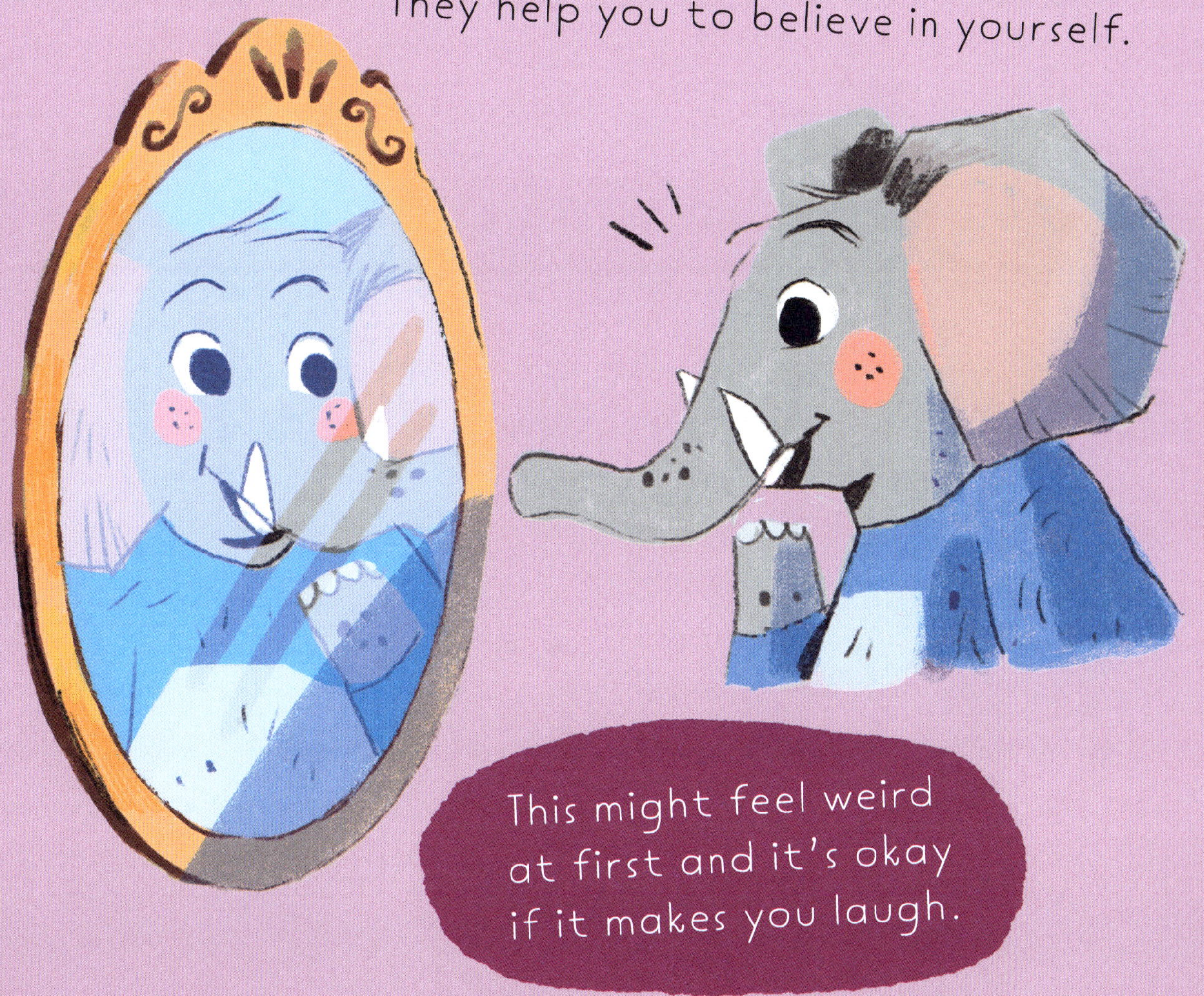

How do you feel after speaking to yourself so nicely? Does it make you smile and feel more confident?

Next week choose another one and have another go.

Speak up

Speaking up can help you get you what you need.

In class if you put your hand up and say 'I don't understand', your teacher can explain again.

If you tell a friend to stop taking your crayons, they will know you don't like it.

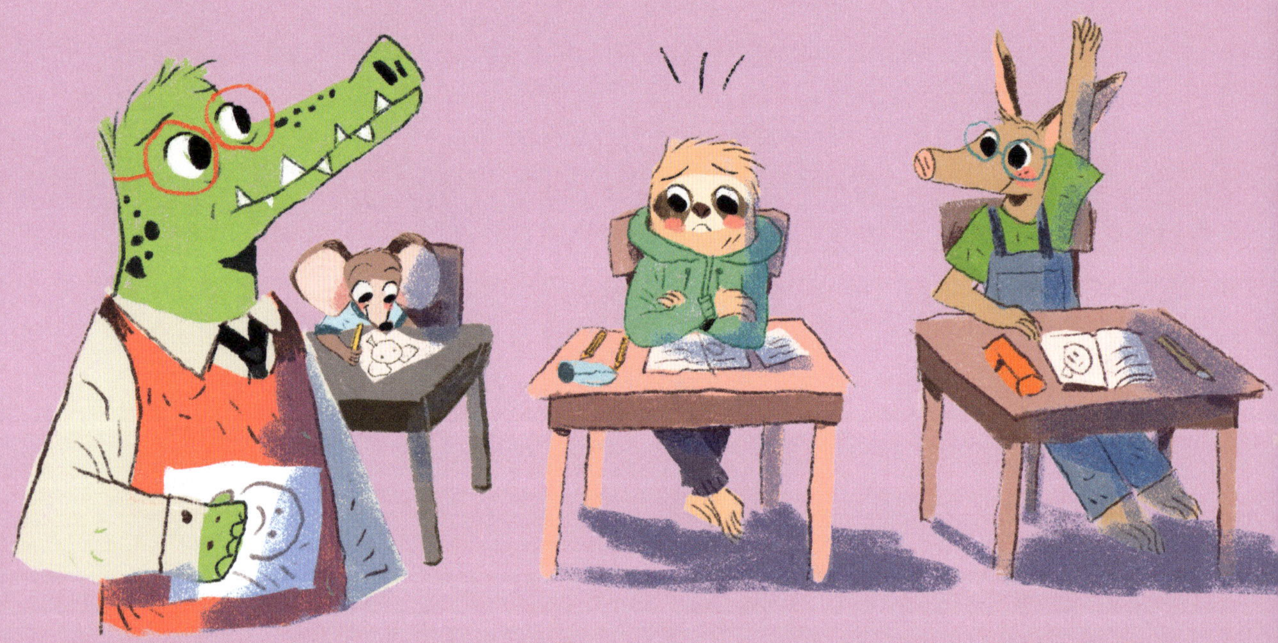

It might feel hard to speak up if you are shy, but it is important people hear what you have to say, and it is a good way to solve problems.

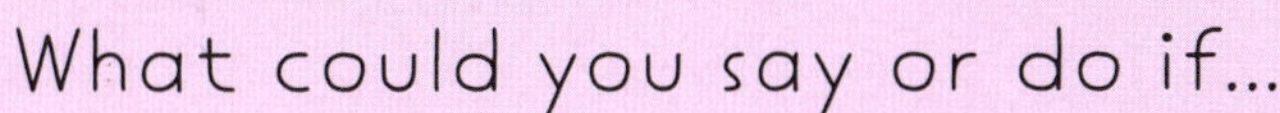

What could you say or do if...

your sister keeps breaking your toy?

someone takes the book you were reading?

you feel left out of a game?

you don't hear what your teacher says?

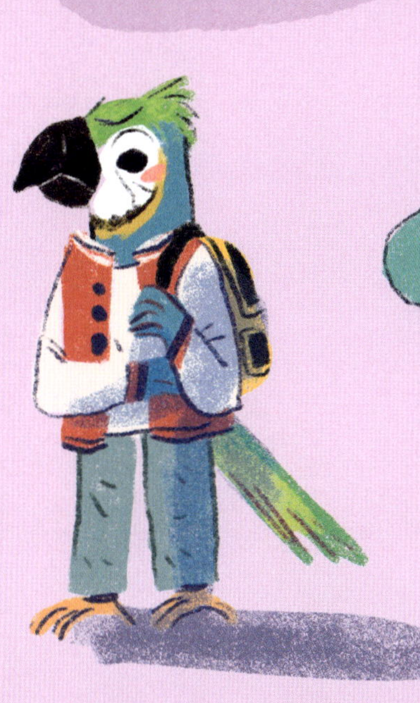

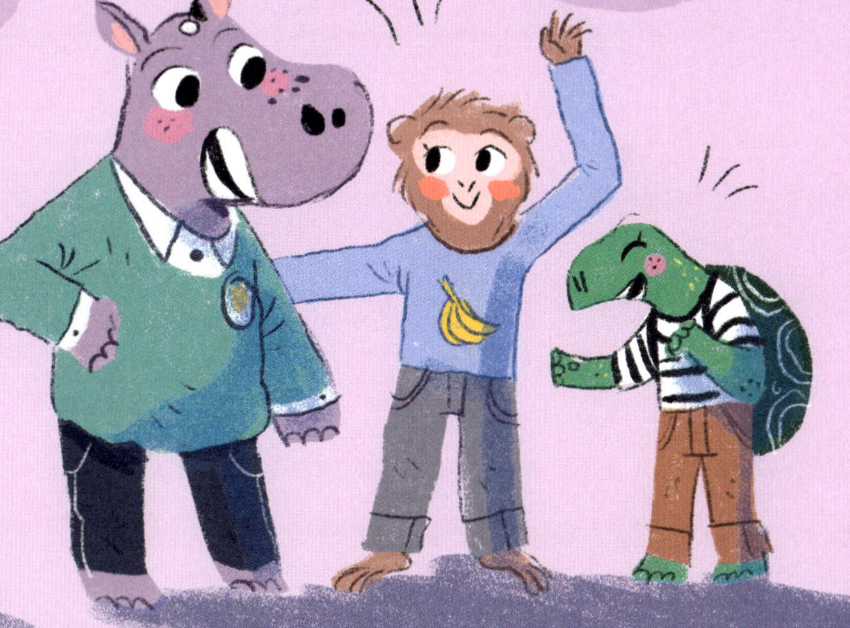

Can you act this out with a grown-up?

Remember, always use a clear, calm voice to ask for what you need. If someone doesn't listen to you, try telling someone else.

The more you practise speaking up the easier it will get.

Draw a confidence rocket

When you are confident you feel good about yourself. You trust people will like you and that you can cope with difficult things, like going to a new school and making new friends.

If you think about all the great things about you, it can help you feel more confident.

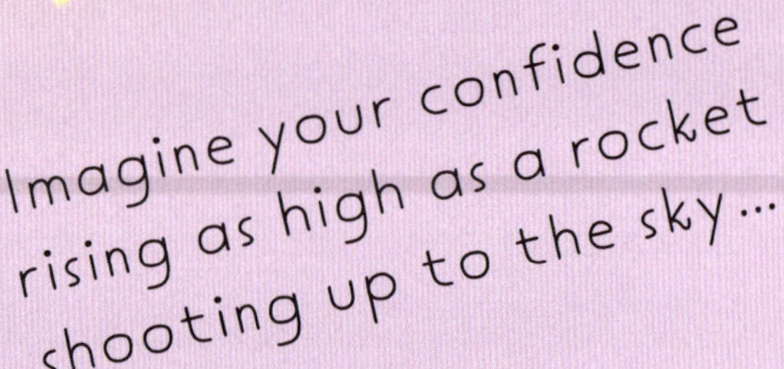

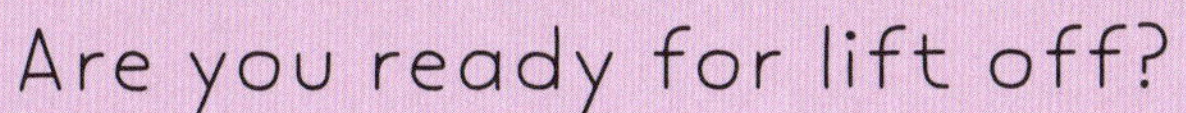
Are you ready for lift off?

Can you name...?

3 people who like you a lot

2 nice things about you

1 thing you are really good at

Blast off!

Can you draw a picture of a rocket shooting up to the stars?

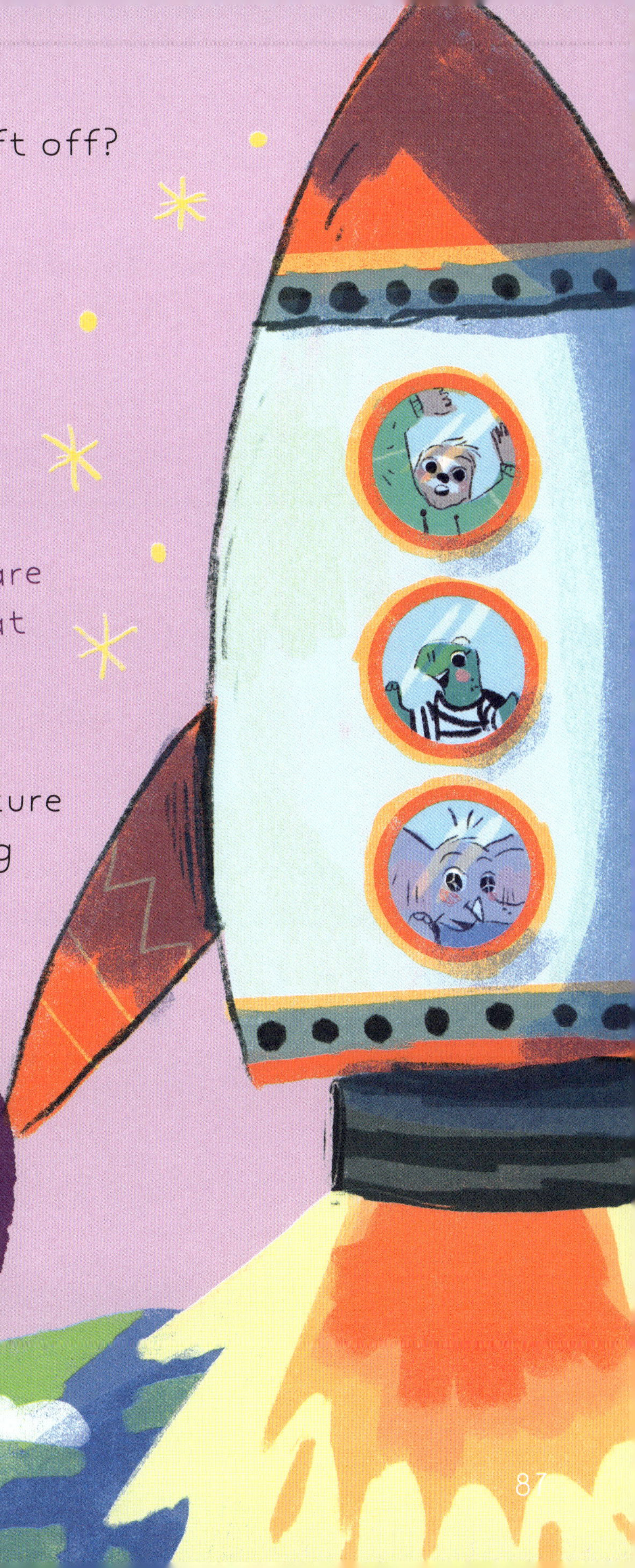

If your confidence ever needs to rise just look at your rocket drawing and answer the 3, 2, 1 questions again.

Become a superhero

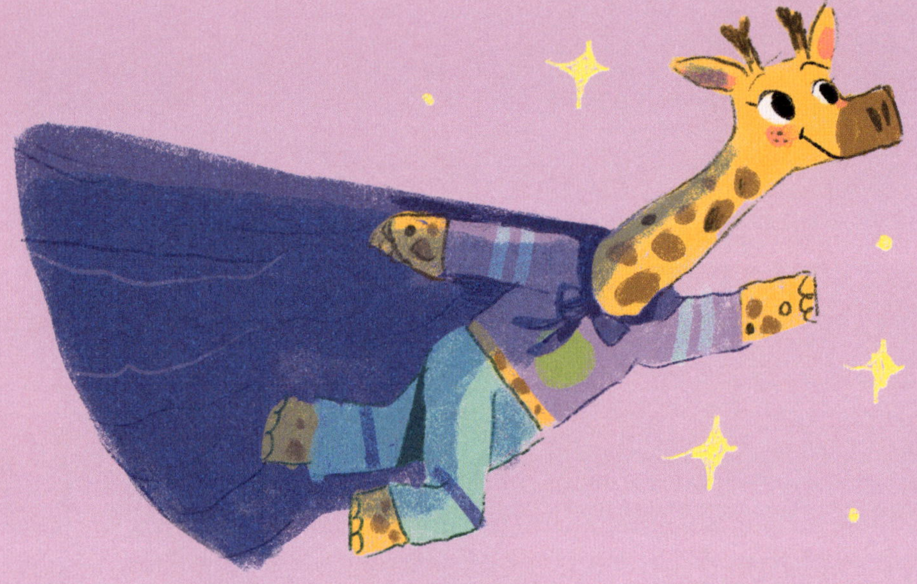

Being brave doesn't mean you aren't scared. Being brave means that you might feel scared, but you give something a try anyway.

It can help to pretend you are wearing a cape, like your favourite superhero, when you need to be brave.

What superpowers would it give you?

What fear would you face?

Have a go at drawing or making your own cape of courage and decorate it with stickers and felt tip pens, like Gilly Giraffe has done.

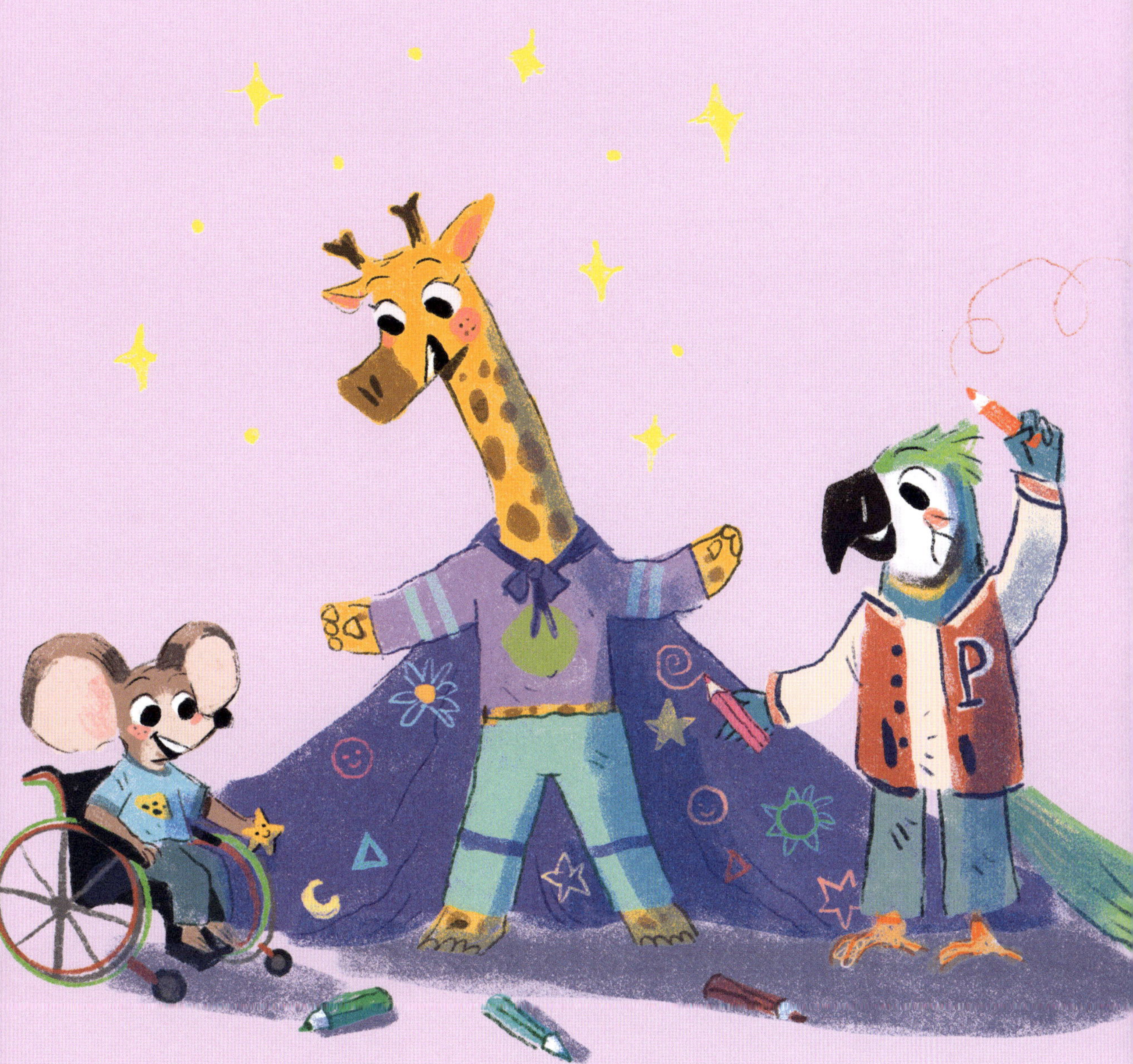

Face your fears

Some fears are real and helpful - like being scared of sharp scissors.

Some fears aren't real or helpful. Tiny spiders or the dark won't hurt you, you may just think they are scary.

Thoughts aren't always true.

Do you have a fear you would like to get over?

Let's have a go.

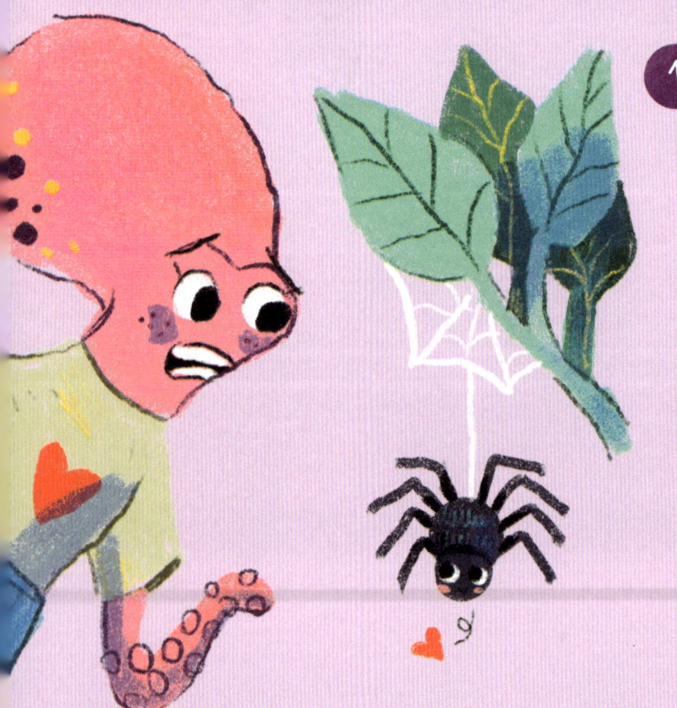

1. Turn your fear into a goal and write or draw it in the middle of a page.

   If you are scared of spiders your goal might be....

   Look at a spider without screaming.

2 Come up with lots of ideas that could help you and add them to your paper. Include actions that get you used to your scary thing.

Look at spider videos.

Draw a spider.

Get a spider cuddly toy.

Read a book on spiders.

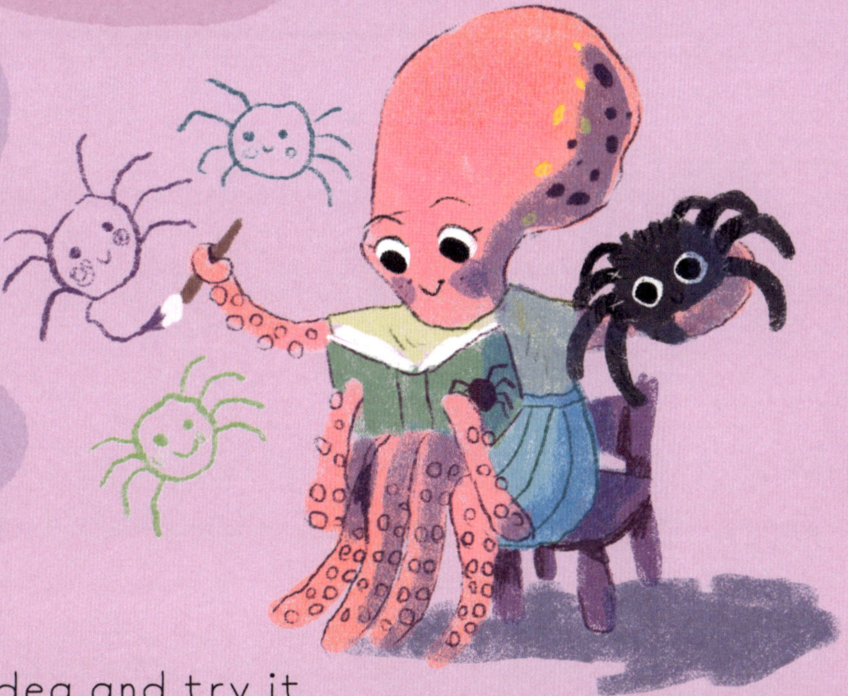

3 Pick one idea and try it. Then pick another.

Each time you do something to face your fear you will feel braver. You will soon reach your goal.

For grown-ups

Encourage your child to face their fear them by adopting a positive attitude and sharing practical suggestions.

Amazing you!

If you think about what you can't do, it can make you feel weak.

If you think about what you can do, it can make you feel strong. Feeling strong helps you to try new and hard things.

Point to each part of your body and say out loud what it can do.

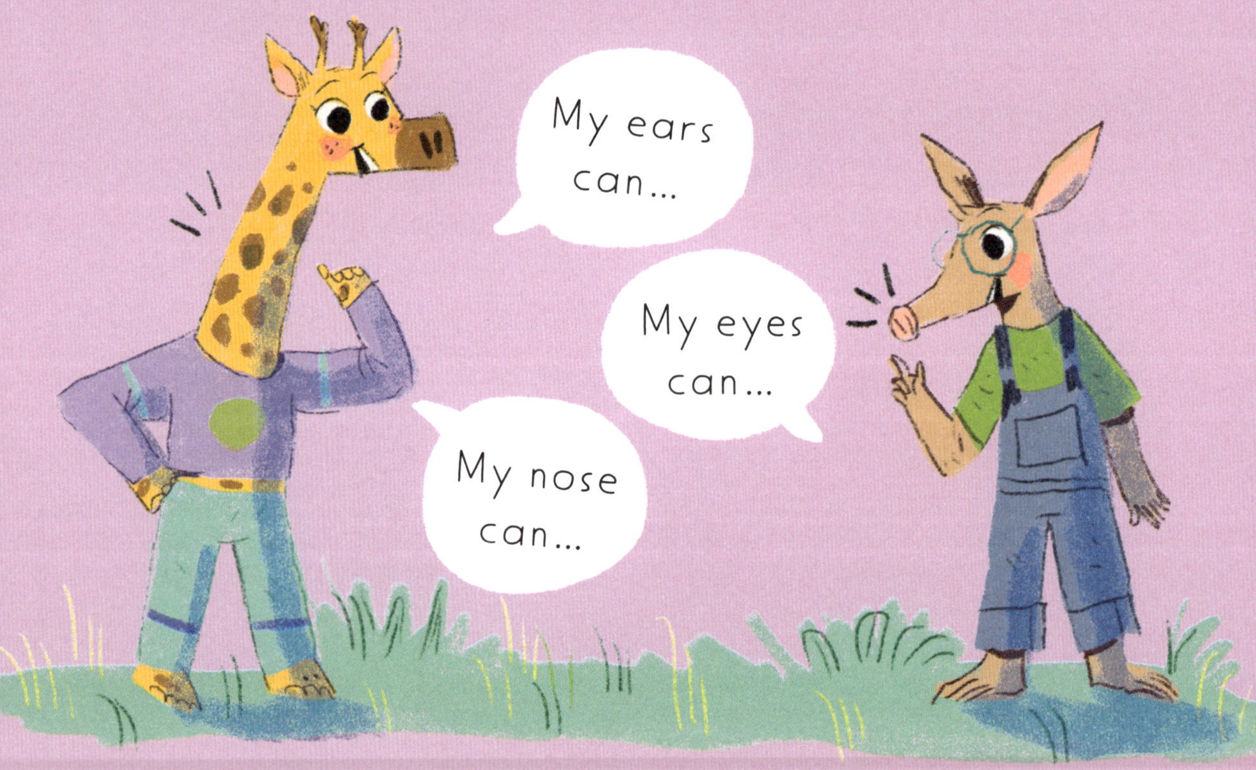

And go all the way down to your toes.

Now point to your brain - what are all the incredible things it can do?

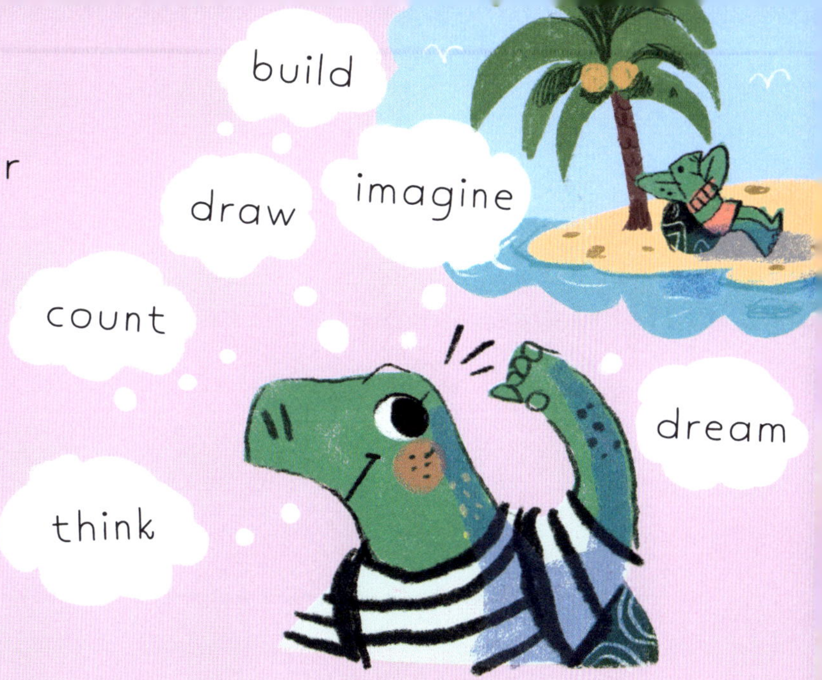

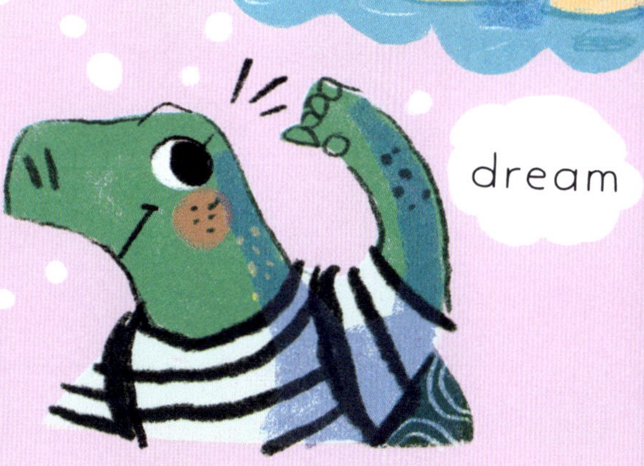

You are amazing!

Now raise your arms up in a V sign as if you had won a race. This is a good way to celebrate yourself.

Don't forget other people's bodies and brains might work differently to yours. And that's okay. Everyone is amazing in their own wonderful way.

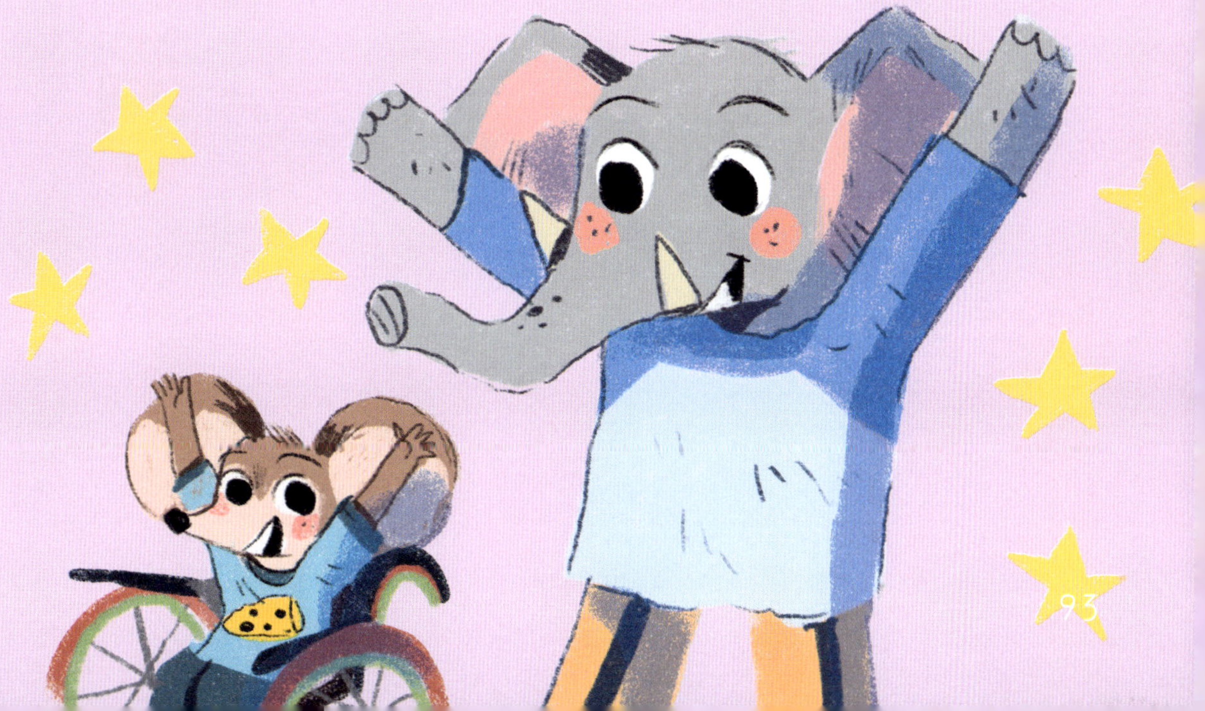

Do the cushion walk

When things go wrong some people get sad and won't try again. They tell themselves they 'can't do it'.

But if instead of saying 'I can't do it' they said 'I can't do it yet' it would encourage them to have another go.

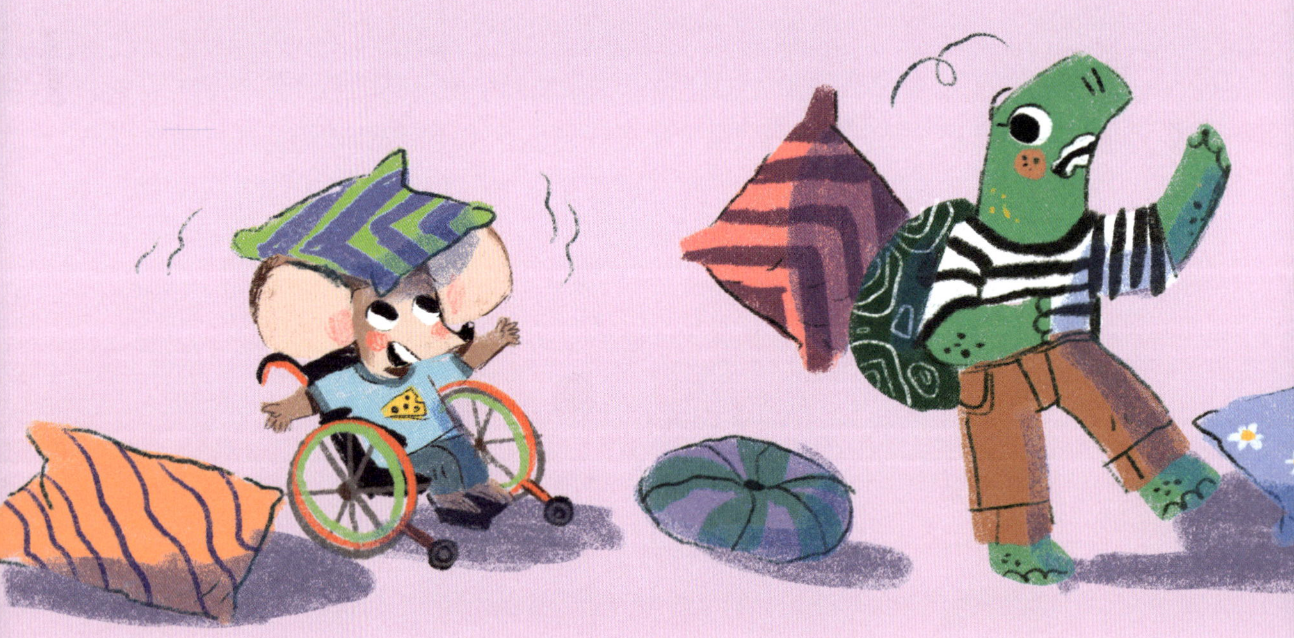

Try this:

Walk across the room with a cushion on your head. When it falls off, try hopping across the room. When it falls off, just pick it up and try again.

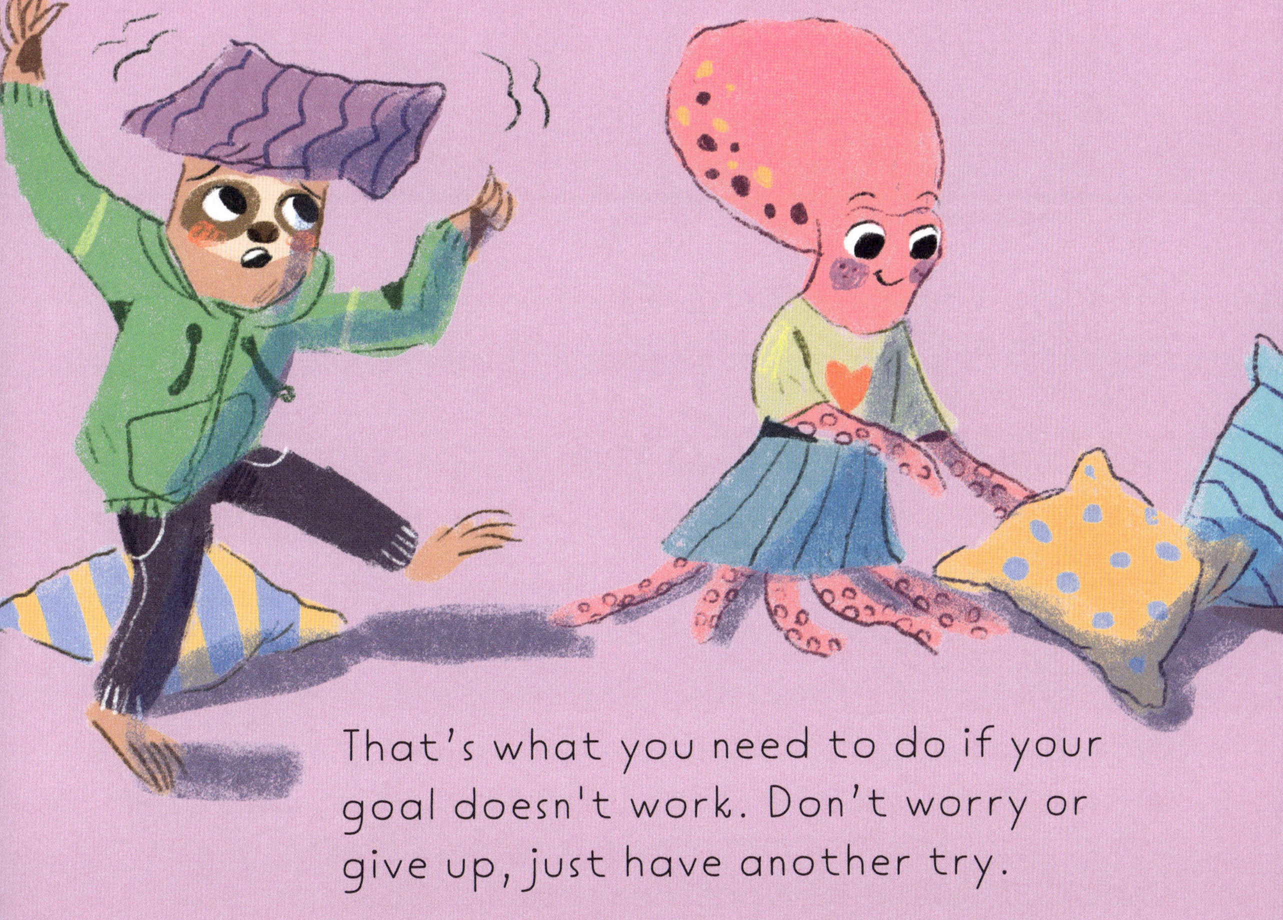

That's what you need to do if your goal doesn't work. Don't worry or give up, just have another try.

Things don't have to be perfect for them to be fun and worth doing.

For grown-ups

If your child says 'I can't do it' model adding 'yet' to the end of their sentence and don't forget to use it yourself when tempted to say 'I can't'.

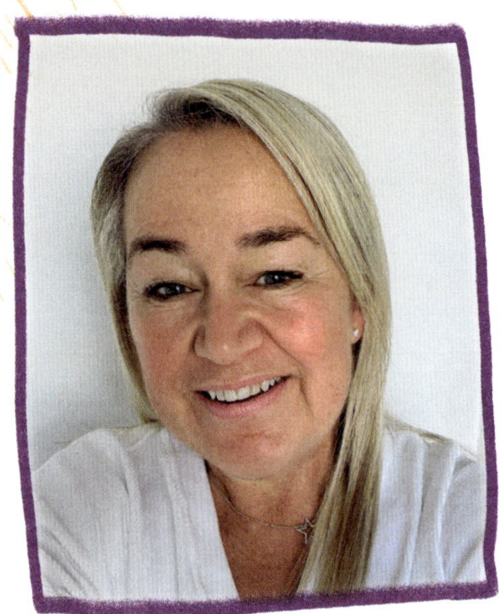

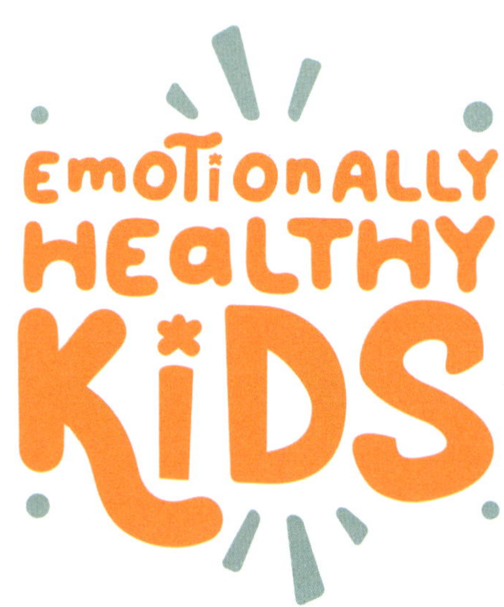

My name is Becky Goddard-Hill and I am a children's wellbeing author, psychotherapist and founder of Emotionally Healthy Kids.

As a former Social Worker specialising in childcare, I ran training in many areas of children's emotional development.

Supporting children through life's challenges, managing anger and developing better self-esteem are key aspects of my work.

Just as we support children's academic learning it is also vital to support their social and emotional learning, and this is the aim of How I feel. Children need our support in these areas to develop robust emotional health and wellbeing and to increase their emotional intelligence.

I hope the activities in this book prove useful in providing the tools to help and encourage children from a young age. We all want our children to be emotionally healthy kids... let's give them a guiding hand.

You can find some helpful videos and resources for parents, carers and teachers at **collins.co.uk/howifeel**